CHALLENGING STRESS, BURNOUT AND RUST-OUT

CHALLENGING STRESS, BURNOUT AND RUST-OUT

Finding Balance in Busy Lives

Teena J. Clouston

Jessica Kingsley *Publishers*
London and Philadelphia

Cartoons (Figures 5.4–5.8 and 6.1) and drawings (Figures 4.1 and 4.2) by Peter Cronin

First published in 2015
by Jessica Kingsley Publishers
73 Collier Street
London N1 9BE, UK
and
400 Market Street, Suite 400
Philadelphia, PA 19106, USA

www.jkp.com

Copyright Teena J. Clouston © 2015

Front cover image source: iStockphoto.

Library of Congress Cataloging in Publication Data
A CIP catalog record for this book is available from the Library of Congress
Clouston, Teena J.
  Challenging stress, burnout and rust-out : finding balance in busy lives / Teena J. Clouston.
    pages cm
  Includes bibliographical references and index.
  ISBN 978-1-84905-406-5 (alk. paper)
  1. Burn out (Psychology) 2. Stress management. 3. Lifestyles--Psychological aspects. I. Title.
  BF481.C573 2015
  155.9'042--dc23
                            2015008373

British Library Cataloguing in Publication Data
A CIP catalogue record for this book is available from the British Library

ISBN 978 1 84905 406 5
eISBN 978 0 85700 786 5

Printed and bound in the United States

For my parents

The old lady thought with the wings of a dove,
Quietly, silently, misty and grey.
Fetch me a raindrop from over the hill
That has trapped the rays of the sun.
Give me a cloud that holds flour and corn
And a mouse's tail curled up by the sun.
Swallows' wings I can sew to my heels
To catch the years I've sung.
Spin me a spider's web, silken and fine,
Pearled with crystal dew.
Raise me an echo, clear from the hill
To rouse the love I knew.
Make me a mirror of melted snow,
Pure from the roof of the world.
Hold me a chariot of silver and gold,
To ride the years to come.
Lend me an arrow and a bow
To tap nectar from the sun.

Thomas O. Dodge

ACKNOWLEDGEMENTS

Thanks to Peter Cronin for unerring support and the drawings and cartoons. www.petercronin.org

CONTENTS

LIST OF FIGURES, BOXES AND TABLES

PREFACE

What is this Book About?

This book, as the title suggests, is about *life balance*. That term can have many different meanings to many different people, so to begin with let me clarify that in this text it is about having a sense of *personal fulfillment and harmony* in everyday life that leads to *health and wellbeing*. This should, of course, be achievable for all of us, but strangely enough, this kind of experience is quite alien to many in modern Western economies and has become a rather elusive concept, almost utopian in its absence, and is something that many of us seek, yet cannot find.

The first part of this book explores why a sense of balance has become so idealized and difficult to achieve in contemporary life and it takes two approaches to this. First, using case studies and examples, it discusses the challenges of finding balance in everyday life when we are *overworked* and/ or *over-busy* and considers why we view *paid work* as a separate domain (area or sphere of activity) from the rest of life, including *unpaid work*: the essential or obligatory jobs and tasks we do everyday like domestic chores, caring for others and often, especially if you are unemployed or retired, community support or voluntary activities that can become expected or required by others in your everyday 'doing'. These kinds of *purposive* activities are often the things that keep us busy and dominate our daily routines.

Second, and this is an integral concept of the book, it describes how life balance is multidimensional and far more complicated than work–life balance theories suggest in their diametrical opposition to the domains of paid work and the rest of life. In order to capture this complexity of life balance I suggest we think about it in terms of a dance of time and energy between doing, being, belonging and becoming activities. These dimensions describe the different types of things we do every day: the purposive, goal-oriented 'doing' activities, the reflective and meaningful 'being' activities and the 'belonging' relationships and connections we hold with others in both the social and natural environment, all of which are necessary to achieve 'becoming' who we truly are and want to be in life.

WHY IS LIFE BALANCE A PROBLEM IN MODERN LIFE?

Well, first of all, it is not difficult for everyone, but in most Western economies productivity and growth are the ultimate achievement; in basic terms, these kinds of cultures want to make money and spend it to stimulate growth and create wealth. In order to achieve this, most have fiscal policies based on the principles of *neoliberal capitalism*, which, in basic terms, uses people as workers to resource the cycle of production by exchanging time and energy for money and promoting models of consumerism and consumption through global markets. In order to stimulate growth and activity, neoliberalism has deregulated these markets and increased the power of the organizations that function in them. At the same time it has reduced or eliminated the welfare state and eroded workers' rights by disempowering trade unions. As a result the 'market' has become almost omnipotent in its practice, and where the working person is part of the cycle of production, this is not good news: the drive for growth *uses* or *consumes* the employee's time and energy to best advantage and can be greedy in the use of these resources; as people have limited power to challenge this practice, so they can become pressured, stressed and exhausted, and their lives can become seriously imbalanced by the demands of the paid workplace.

Now this may seem bad enough, but neoliberalism has a few other principles that can make this use of human resources, that is *your* time and energy, even worse. First, neoliberalism promotes *individualism* which means that the individual (you) is valued more than the collective or whole (family, community, society) but also places the individual person (you), as *responsible for his or her own actions* and therefore culpable for *all* decisions made in life. In terms of life balance, this means the choice and decisions *you make* to achieve life balance and the intended and unintended consequences that occur as a result of *your* choices are your *own* responsibility, and have nothing to do with how much the workplace or significant others demand of you. Moreover, in the paid workplace, workers are subject to *greater levels of scrutiny* and *control* in order to ensure that this notion of individual responsibility is fully implemented. Those who *do not* participate in paid work, whether this is due to other demands on time and energy like caring commitments, or a lack of job opportunities, ill health, disability or even retirement, do not escape this sense of carrying the can for choices made and are made to feel accountable for their unemployed state and any repercussions this might entail.

Second, because neoliberalism functions on the principle of consumerism in *global markets*, competition is higher and more aggressive, because there is more choice for consumers (you). When competition is high and markets insistent, the capturing of consumers (you) becomes paramount and the pressure to make you spend is intensified. For your part, as a consumer, you are expected to engage more with markets to increase the profit margins and maintain a competitive edge through buying more stuff to increase the wealth of your nation.

Of course, being unemployed can be a very challenging place to be in this kind of fiscal model because if you are *not* working, and therefore *not* earning, you are not spending as much as consumers *should be* to maximize growth; consequently, you are not as valued as those who can promote the cycles of consumption and productivity. We overcome this in a couple of ways: depending on your personality and social circumstances you may become despondent and feel disenfranchised from society, or alternatively, you may start filling up your 'spare' time to be as busy as you can be by doing unpaid but socially worthy or obligatory tasks to make yourself seem useful. According to Hochschild (2008, p.89) this need for busyness is almost like a drug, 'the opiate of the masses'; a necessary evil in our everyday lives to achieve a sense of self-worth.

Using case studies and examples, I will show in this book how paid work can be greedy in terms of our personal resources of time and energy and can cause work–life imbalance, resulting in stress and exhaustion. I will also consider how the drive to be over-busy, whether you are in paid work or not, can have similar effects. I will identify how these kinds of practices promote doing obligatory and purposive tasks over all others and, moreover, can steal time and energy resources needed for other activities in life, like family commitments, including caring and loving relationships, social and leisure pursuits, community participation, altruistic endeavours, thinking and reflective time and, perhaps most insidiously and frequently hidden, time to be in the natural environment and to do *personally meaningful* (usually the things you *freely choose* to do and *enjoy*) *activities* or *occupations* (occupations in the context of this book literally means all the activities you do every day as a way of spending or 'occupying' your time). Consequently, although the book does use the stories and experiences of a group of working professionals to convey some of its message, it is not exclusively for those people who feel worked out (exhausted; worn down; burnt out) as a result of just paid work. It is for all of us who are searching for a greater sense of balance and personal meaning in life.

KEY MESSAGES IN THE BOOK

The book is premised on seven key principles.

PRINCIPLE ONE: BALANCE EQUALS WELLBEING

The first and the most simple principle is the belief that people need to find a sense of balance, fulfillment or harmony in their lives in order to achieve a sense of wellbeing in everyday life. This principle advocates that living in balance is a central tenet of wellbeing in everyday life.

PRINCIPLE TWO: WE SPEND TOO MUCH TIME 'DOING' THINGS

The second principle is based on the fact that we can use *too much* of our personal resources of *time and energy* in *obligatory* things and not enough in more restful and recuperative '*being*' types of pursuits or those focused on our sense of belonging and becoming who we truly want to be. This kind of over-emphasis on doing obligatory activities or being busy all of the time is endemic in Western economies and actually creates a pervasive state of imbalance in life. For example, the paid work domain has been commonly highlighted as the culprit in taking too much of our time and energy, which we, as a result of social norms, are often complicit in, either by feeling coerced by others, or indeed freely giving over our time and energy to that activity, even though we know it is detrimental to other life domains, including the home, the family, our social and leisure pursuits, community participation, spending time in nature, and other more restive, recuperative or reflective occupations. The problem with this kind of lifestyle is that the sharing and/or reconciling of time and energy across a variety of different activities is essential to a sense of wellbeing in everyday life and this is challenged or constrained because variety and choice in daily activities are rather elusive when paid work, or the need to be seen to be busy all of the time, predominates as a social norm; in essence, we lose variety, which is the spice of life.

PRINCIPLE THREE: DOING TOO MUCH IS DETRIMENTAL TO WELLBEING

The third principle identifies that the outcome of this overwork and over-busyness is that we often feel *overburdened, overcommitted, exhausted* and *stressed*. This can lead to *burnout*, which is an emotional, psychological and physical state evidenced by exhaustion and chronic stress or '*rust-out*', marked by a lack of engagement in activities, which can be identified by apathy, withdrawal and disinterest in our everyday lives. Rust-out is closely associated with demotivation and can exist as a result of too many mundane, routine type activities, or a lack of personally meaningful or challenging pursuits because we lack a sense of engagement in life. I will define these terms in Chapter 1 (but also see the glossary at the end of this book) and talk about these troubling states of dis-ease and why they occur in Chapter 4.

PRINCIPLE FOUR: PERSONALLY MEANINGFUL ACTIVITIES ARE ESSENTIAL TO LIFE BALANCE

The fourth principle maintains that at least some of the activities we do in everyday life should include those that are *personally meaningful* i.e. *freely chosen* and *spiritual* or *emotionally fulfilling* and not just be focused on obligatory tasks all of the time. This does not mean to say that everything we do needs to have a sense of personal meaning for us, but that some, or at least one, of the things we do in everyday life should. Why, you may ask, is this important? Well if you feel that some activities (and paid work can fall into this category) give you a sense of *personal meaning* then you tend to *engage* with it. If you *engage* with an activity then you are inclined to focus on it and give it your *full attention* when you are doing it. Csikszentmihalyi (1997) has called this kind of focused attention 'psychic energy', and believes the use of this kind of energy can facilitate a sense of *flow*, or full absorption and involvement in an activity. When in this sense of flow, we can often find time slows down because we are so involved with the activity we can *engage* with it to the exclusion of those disruptive thoughts and feelings like that constant white noise or mental chatter that can plague our more mundane tasks. This sense of being at one or fully engaged with an activity can be facilitated in the active 'doing' as well as the more reflective 'being' types of activities and, by inducing a sense of enjoyment and pleasure in life, can create and sustain a sense of harmony and promote wellbeing; 'The present moment is filled with joy and happiness. If you are attentive, you will see it' (Hanh 1991a, p.21).

PRINCIPLE FIVE: LIFE BALANCE IS COMPLICATED

The fifth principle is that life balance is not two-dimensional or linear, as in the notion of the two arms of a scale that can be balanced, but rather that it is *multidimensional,* marked by the interaction of *doing, being, becoming and belonging activities.* These create a complex and interconnected web of *relational* (having interconnected relationships) forces that act upon one another creating a *dynamic* (constantly changing; adaptive) and *synergic* (something more than its separate parts) dance of time and energy to create the rhythm of life. This means that life balance does not follow simple rules and the notion that stability can be precisely found at one point of equilibrium (like balancing one domain with the others as in the work–life balance scenario) is far too simple.

PRINCIPLE SIX: RECONCILE RATHER THAN COMPROMISE LIFE CONFLICTS

This brings us to the sixth principle. Thinking about life balance in terms of a complex adaptive web shifts the perspective of addressing it from trying to control balance in different life domains, say for example, by changing time and energy use in one arm of the scale (called work) to get it in balance with the other arm of the scale (called life), to enhancing their capacity to coexist in mutually satisfying ways. This, I suggest, can be achieved by *reconciling* the conflicts between different domains and dimensions of life rather than *compromising* non-obligatory or *personally meaningful* activities to achieve those considered to be socially obligatory.

PRINCIPLE SEVEN: SEEK MEANING, NOT PERFORMANCE, IN LIFE

Finally, the seventh principle of the book advocates we challenge the *performance orientation* we live by in neoliberal Western economies and re-orient ourselves to focus on the meaning of life. This may seem a rather big statement, particularly when socio-cultural-political drivers promote the former; but it is important to remember that in non-linear systems such as a complex, interconnected web, small actions can have enormous consequences and that means you, as a part of the web of life balance, *can* make changes to how you live your everyday life balance and that this *can* have a positive outcome, not only for yourself but for your family, your workplace, your community, your social networks and, through participation in it and care of it, even your natural environment. We have to learn to live in harmony not only with ourselves, our families and communities but also with our planet, something Hanh (1991b, p.226) has called our 'interbeing' or 'dependent co-arising' with the rest of life.

WHERE DO THE IDEAS IN THE BOOK COME FROM?

I have mentioned that case studies are used to describe some of the principles in the book. The examples noted in the text are taken from a study that explored the life balance of a professional group called occupational therapists. Occupational therapists are specialists in health and social care and tend to work in these fields. In the United Kingdom (UK), where the study took place, these kinds of organizations fall into the public sector, which means they are not for profit and can be freely accessed.

OVERVIEW OF THE BOOK

The book is divided into two parts.

PART 1

Part one introduces the theory of life balance and some of the barriers to achieving it in modern life. It describes the experiences of stress, exhaustion, burnout and the lack of engagement, or *rust-out*, that people can experience as a result of being overworked and/or over-busy in their everyday lives and explains how this can lead to a lack of *balance* and *personal meaning* in life.

Chapter 1 considers the question 'what *is* life balance?', identifies how life balance is linked to *wellbeing* and sets the scene for the book.

Chapter 2 explores *why* we are driven to do too much in modern life and, using examples, considers some of the dilemmas that can occur as a result of our pervasive, overworked and over-busy cultures.

Chapter 3 looks at the conflicts between activities that are classified as *obligatory* and those that are categorized as *non-obligatory* and considers *how* that influences everyday life balance. As part of this it looks at the stereotypical ideas about gender and the division of both paid and unpaid labor.

Chapter 4 looks at the physiology of the human stress response and *how* that can influence the outcomes of living imbalanced lifestyles, including *stress, burnout* and *rust-out*.

PART 2

Part 2 is more practically focused and offers some techniques, strategies and ideas to address imbalance in our everyday lives.

Chapter 5 explores strategies aimed at managing *stress* levels and becoming aware of your thoughts. Thinking can be a very potent tool in underpinning how you feel about your life balance, causing either stress, worry and tension or, conversely, a more positive and relaxed outlook on life. The chapter explores how different personality types can impact on how you perceive and respond to your life balance.

Chapter 6 introduces the techniques of *mindfulness* and considers how these can help with finding balance in busy lives. It explains how we can address the speeded up sense of time we experience in Western life by offering the opportunity to live in the moment and appreciate time as it unfolds. Learning these techniques helps to wake us up from our *mindless* state and this assists in facilitating engagement in life activities.

Chapter 7 talks about the importance of spending time and energy in *personally meaningful activities* and looks at strategies that can help you create the space, time and energy for activities that *you feel* are important to you. These may not necessarily be socially classed as purposeful because they do not generate money, but in fact, for wellbeing, these activities are the most important to have in your repertoire of daily life. Consequently, they *do* have a real purpose in terms of life balance because they facilitate *fulfillment* and are *engaging* as well as *meaningful*.

Chapter 8 looks at how the *workplace* and *labor market* could change to provide a better and more supportive place to be in terms of achieving *life balance* and *wellbeing*. It considers how we can establish a sense of personal autonomy over life balance, even in cultures that intensify imbalance and in situations where others have more power than us.

Chapter 9 considers how we can think about life balance in a more interconnected, resilient and sustainable way and summarizes the key messages and strategies found in the book in terms of living a balanced lifestyle.

PART 1

UNDERSTANDING LIFESTYLE BALANCE AND ITS LINK TO WELLBEING

CHAPTER 1
WHAT IS LIFE BALANCE?

INTRODUCTION

Asking the question 'what *is* life balance?' is an interesting one, because there are a variety of different views on it. As described in the Preface, this book sees life balance as a complex and interconnected web that includes the social and natural worlds in which we live, which link together to achieve a meaningful sense of personal fulfillment, harmony and wellbeing in life.

Whilst this kind of complexity and vision of life balance may be relatively unique, some of the concepts, such as the need for spending time in meaningful activities and the integration of life domains (especially paid work and life) are not. These kinds of perspectives are found in a variety of diverse theoretical backgrounds such as occupational science (the theory and knowledge base of the profession of occupational therapy), sociology, psychology and feminism, to mention but a few of the interested parties.

Occupational science encapsulates its theories of life balance into a philosophy it calls *occupational balance*. This philosophy pertains that wellbeing can only be found in a personally meaningful balance across a variety of different life domains. For others, the term *work–life balance* is frequently used as a euphemism for balancing the demands of paid work with family commitments, thus excluding a more complex vision of life's myriad activities; whilst personal choice and preference are considered in their ideas, personal meaning is less clearly articulated than in the notions of occupational balance.

Strangely enough, although these various theories do differ in perspectives, they do also share some common themes, so to simplify for the reader I am going to discuss them under the two broad headings of first, work–life balance and second, occupational balance and personal meaning, because this will facilitate discussion of both the differences and the commonalities in the ideas held about life balance.

WORK–LIFE BALANCE THEORIES

Work–life balance theories, as the name suggests, tend to be concerned with the balance between the paid work domain and, specifically in this context, family and caring commitments. At the most basic level, the theory goes that people cross the borders (Clark 2000) between the domain of paid work and the home, trying to meet the demands to participate meaningfully in both, but are challenged in achieving this because they call on the same pot of time and energy reserves. This suggests that supplies are insufficient to meet demands and begs the question, why are we doing too much?

The idea of conflict or tension between paid work and the home domain is, in many ways, quite culturally specific, shaped by the fiscal models of Western neoliberal capitalism. As discussed in the introduction, neoliberalism is a branch of capitalism that drives economic growth and productivity through global markets (consumerism and consumption of resources); that, in turn, intensifies pressures in paid work and this means workers become ever more busy and have even less time for activities outside of paid work, including the essential family domain, fuelling the conflict between these two critical aspects of daily life.

Now whilst this conflict may, at first, seem surmountable (for example through support networks) the problem is that this same social structure intensifying working practices also promotes the adult labor model, which means that people of working age, irrespective of their caring responsibilities, are expected to participate in paid work. Now again, this seems fair: if we can work, why not? But when you consider a third driver expects an *ethically* and *morally* sound investment in family life, you have to begin to wonder how all that can be achieved effectively by one person.

Under these circumstances, it is notable that neoliberal labor markets *do* recognize reciprocity or mutuality between life domains, because they maintain that moves to increase flexibility in the workplace are there to *support* the conflicts employees experience from the home into the workplace and vice versa. However, in reality this kind of market concerns itself only with the former, and the overflow of pressures from paid work into the home is less considered. Thus flexible working is more a tool of employee *efficiency* rather than one to promote employee *wellbeing* (we will return to this point throughout the book). By the nature of the need for growth and productivity, neoliberalism favors participation in paid work above all other life domains, and consequently *creates* work–life imbalance. Sadly, as a consequence of global markets, this kind of fiscal and human productivity model is no longer exclusively a Western phenomenon and has become an approach applied to economies and labor markets across the world. This leads us nicely to the categories of occupational balance, personal meaning and choice.

OCCUPATIONAL BALANCE, PERSONAL MEANING AND CHOICE

Theories promoting occupational balance, meaning and choice believe that participation in meaningful activities and a balance between *multiple life domains* (differing from the two-dimensional notion of paid work and family/caring found in work–life balance theories) can promote a sense of identity and enhance personal wellbeing: 'To live is to enfold multiple occupations [or activities] which provide enjoyment, payment, personal identity and more' (Townsend 1997, p.19).

Debates over the number and complexity of life activities (or occupations) proliferate, recognizing myriad ideologies stretching from the simplistic triads of self-care, productivity and leisure common in occupational science (e.g. Creek 2003) and the work, rest and play scenario made famous by the Mars bar confectionary advert, to the more complex, which includes research by Cummins (1996) identifying over 170 life domains, including paid work, financial resources, leisure, dwelling and neighborhood, family, friendships, social participation and health, to mention but a few.

At this juncture it is perhaps important to note that whilst I do make reference to different domains of life and activities or occupations in the book, using terms such as paid work, family, domestic, leisure and social pursuits to clarify points, I will introduce and promote a model found in occupational science literature that avoids the categorization of life activities in this way by describing life as the purposive or active *doing* types of occupations in life (like paid work); the *being* activities, which are those that are more restive, recuperative and appreciative in nature; the *becoming* activities that promote self-actualizing and self-identity; and the *belonging* activities, those that are *relational* in nature or create a sense of *belonging*. I will describe these categories in more detail later in the chapter.

WHAT DO WE MEAN BY PERSONAL MEANING?

Theoretical underpinnings in occupational science also identify a specific interest in the *personal meaning* and *subjective experience* of the individual. Explicitly, these investigate what the value and meaning of activities (or occupations) are for the individual and a belief that personal wellbeing, balance and harmony are found through creating the space and time to incorporate these key occupations into everyday life.

In a similar vein, sociologists Thompson and Bunderson (2001) have argued that the *subjective meaning* people assign to activities is imperative to finding a sense of balance because when these preferences match or are *congruent* with our personal interests and who we want to be, so they promote a personal sense of self (a congruent and coherent self) and are identity-affirming because we are living our lives the way that we want to, feel happy about and therefore gain personal *fulfillment, harmony* and *wellbeing* from.

Following on from this kind of thinking, theorists like Csikszentmihalyi (1997; 2002) (mentioned in the introduction) identified the value of engagement and using *psychic energy*, that is, giving one's full attention and focus to an activity to facilitate personal pleasure, fulfillment and subsequently wellbeing in life.

The problem with these theories is that to spend time in activities that achieve a sense of personal meaning requires an initial investment of time and energy in order to kick-start the process. This requires surplus energy, initiative and drive, something very hard to find for the exhausted, overworked, over-busy or de-motivated individual who tends to migrate towards the less challenging, passive or mind-numbing pursuits of watching TV, consumerism (shopping or browsing... you know the one... retail therapy), or the virtual worlds of computer games and social media.

If this is not you, how many people do you know that use one or more of these *mindless* (in the sense that you do not have to engage or think) activities in their lives? In this book I argue that achieving and sustaining a *personally meaningful* life balance requires time and energy to be reserved and given to pursuits that are *engaging* and can capture your attention, passion or interest because this can facilitate a sense of creativity, fulfillment, wellbeing and meaning in life. But, as I have already intimated, finding the time and energy to do this in neoliberal market economies is more than a little problematic, and one of those problems is personal choice.

THE QUESTION OF CHOICE

The option to access personal meaningful pursuits raises the question of making choices about what we do or at least the issue of *free choice* in determining how we spend our time. In the development of her *preference theory* sociologist Catherine Hakim has argued that people in affluent market economies have been given greater space to make active choices about how they form a salient work–life balance because of greater flexibility in the workplace; but she also notes that an individualized approach to worker efficiency and a growing sense of personal responsibility for performance in the workplace means:

> Men and women not only gain the freedom to choose their own biography, values and lifestyle, they are forced to make their own decisions because there are no universal certainties or collectively agreed conventions, no fixed models of the good life, as in traditional or early modern industrial societies. (Hakim 2006, p.286)

Now whilst Hakim uses the word 'forced' in terms of people having to make decisions about how they live their lives, and illustrates how neoliberalism has increased uncertainty and consequently vulnerability in the labor market (I will talk about this in depth later), she interestingly suggests that the choices we make about life balance are *freely chosen*. In particular, she describes women as having more choices than men in how they manage paid work and family commitments because they can *choose* to be work-centered (i.e. place work as their most important activity and build a career); to be home-centered (put the home domain as the priority activity; this tends to be the full-time mother or carer but is not exclusively so) or to be *adaptive*, which means that you choose to participate in both paid work and home domains without giving a fixed priority to either. The latter, Hakim (2006) believes, is the most common choice that women make in modern affluent societies. Alternatively, men are described as tending to be relatively homogenous in their decision-making about work and to be generally adopting the more work-focused pattern, because this of course is the traditional patriarchal model of the male breadwinner.

In many ways Hakim's theory is common sense and offers few surprises to those who work in the more affluent of Western economies, but even in these settings choice is on a sliding scale and consequently I cannot agree that the choices we make are necessarily *freely* chosen because these choices are limited by the options available to us in the fabric of the society in which we are embedded. In neoliberal societies the norms expected of all working age adults is to be *in* paid work, to *perform* in paid work and to support fiscal growth or *production*. The problem with this is that this kind of system may offer more choices in terms of when and where we work (because this supports flexible working patterns) but it has done little to accommodate the *relational* or family concept of society, or indeed the concept of individual wellbeing through the sustainable use of the human resources of time and energy; rather, it drives a *performance orientation*.

Of even more concern is that we have known about these pressures for years and yet have done little to address it. Take for example this comment from Adolph Meyer, a psychiatrist practicing in the early 20th-century, who believed that the post-war drive for growth and money was crippling employee wellbeing:

> Our industrialism has created the false, because one-sided, idea of success in production to the point of overproduction… instead of sound economics of a fair and sane distribution of the goods of this world according to need… The man of today has lost the capacity and pride of workmanship and has substituted for it a measure in terms of money; and now money proves to be of uncertain value. (1922, p.8)

This notion of the value of money as paramount, albeit unpredictable in worth, really resonates with contemporary life, especially in light of the 2007–2008 banking crisis from which many countries have still not recovered. Yet, whilst the foundations of neoliberal capitalism were challenged globally by this financial catastrophe, the neoliberal edifice did not topple and it firmly remains as the ultimate fiscal model.

Consequently, I have to question the need for us to be either exclusively work-focused and performance-driven in paid work, or be excessively busy in non-paid activities, in order to earn the self-worth and social capital necessary to succeed or survive in our social networks. I suggest that if this performance orientation was less dominant as a measure of success in

Western economies, we may have more time and energy to build resilient, sustainable, ethically sound family, community and social networks as well as, in a more ecological context, give time and energy to our natural environment. It is, after all, only this kind of use of time and energy that can strengthen our participation in, and sense of belonging to, our social and natural worlds and through that, create a sense of life balance and wellbeing.

LIFE BALANCE AND WELLBEING

Wellbeing is a personal and subjective experience and consequently the actual essence of what exactly wellbeing is remains mutable. However, most definitions tend to agree that wellbeing is a dynamic, fluid sense of self in which the individual feels able to develop their potential, work productively and creatively, fulfill personal goals, achieve a sense of purpose in society, build strong and positive relationships with others, and contribute to their community (Dewe and Kompier 2008).

This definition resonates with the notion of life balance and encompasses some of the issues raised previously as integral to finding life balance, namely, participation in personally meaningful activities; achieving one's potential and personal goals; having a sense of purpose in life; opportunities for creative pursuits; the need for diversity in daily activities (like time for valued relationships, community and social pursuits); and the significance of paid work and/or a productive role and purpose in society.

Pawar (2013) has identified six different dimensions of wellbeing, which fit well with the complex nature of finding a sense of fulfillment and harmony through life balance. These are physical wellbeing, emotional or subjective wellbeing, psychological wellbeing, social wellbeing, ethical wellbeing and spiritual wellbeing. In one sense these separate dimensions are arbitrary, because as you are one interconnected person, body, mind and soul, so wellbeing is, in fact, a holistic phenomenon (see Figure 1.1). But by examining the separate dimensions as Pawar defines them, we do get a better idea of why we feel imbalance in life, and consequently we will look at these definitions here and use them as a tool to understand the link of life balance to wellbeing in the book.

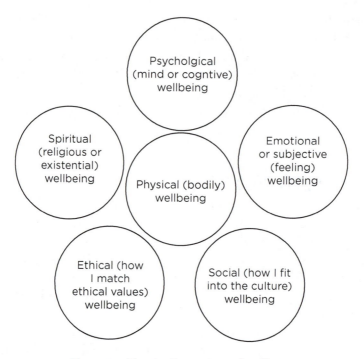

Figure 1.1 The six dimensions of wellbeing

UNDERSTANDING THE DIFFERENT DIMENSIONS OF WELLBEING

The *physical dimension*, as you would expect, refers to bodily health and function; it is how we feel physically. The *emotional* or *subjective* sense of wellbeing refers to the presence of positive emotions as opposed to negative and subsequently, I would suggest, a personal sense of emotional wellbeing as opposed to the opposite, a sense of dis-ease or ill-being in everyday life.

Psychological wellbeing refers to how we think, and importantly includes how we feel about our 'self', namely, our sense of self-acceptance, autonomy, personal growth and personal efficacy or mastery over a variety of life domains. Both the psychological and the emotional/subjective concepts encompass a sense of self-identity, personal congruence and coherence (consistency in knowing who I am) in everyday life.

Social wellbeing is concerned with how we 'fit' with the social environment and is gauged by the contribution we give individually to society; this is about social capital, i.e. social worth and social acceptance by significant others. Notably, what is relevant about this is that one's level of success and self-worth is often a reflection of social values, norms and standards, so is a measure of how one meets the inherent expectations of the relevant social environment. Consequently, this means your sense of life balance and wellbeing is uniquely cultural, defined and shaped by your level of social integration, social contribution, social acceptance and social coherence, specific to your situated context.

Leading on from this *ethical wellbeing*, as you might expect, is about living in an ethically sound way, which, in part, is measured by your congruence with the wider socially acceptable morals, values and behaviors that shape your culture. However, there is an intriguing paradox here in terms of the socially accepted notions of work–life balance in Western concepts of neoliberalism which, in essence, prioritize participation in paid work and actually create the conflict many of us experience between paid work and the rest of our everyday lives: paid work is managed through clock time and participation is frequently measured by presence in the workplace and your *performance orientation* (how hard you work and how much you put into work). This can create ethical dilemmas with home responsibilities because as we dance to the tune of paid work, we are left with little or no option but to try our hardest to fit home commitments around it. Children, or indeed other caring commitments, cannot always be tied up into neat little packets that fit workforce demands; quite the contrary in fact, which brings me straight back to the point of having the opportunity to make meaningful choices in life, because there is little free choice in a world that prioritizes paid work above caring for our children and families, let alone our own personally meaningful interaction with our world. As Gambles, Lewis and Rapoport put it:

> Time and energy to connect with others and give and receive care – as parents, children, lovers and friends, or even time to care for ourselves – are crucial for individual and societal wellbeing. Yet these aspects of life can be increasingly squeezed out by current patterns of paid work or can exclude people with demanding non-paid care responsibilities from much paid work. (2006, p.4)

I will return to these points in Chapter 2.

Finally, *spiritual wellbeing* considers, as indeed you may well think, both the religious and other more existential beliefs that encompass our sense of purpose and/or direction in life: our sense of 'being' in the world.

In essence, this is about who we are and who we want to be or become: our search for *meaning* if you like, and living in congruence with the values we may hold. When considered in this way you could say that spirituality has a both a vertical axis (appreciation of or belief in a transcendent being) and a horizontal one (one's relationships with self, others and the natural environment) (Stoll 1989).

Linking the two dimensions, Muldoon and King (1991, pp.100–101) suggest spirituality 'embodies a certain way of looking at life' and maintain that this 'lived-out vision of life relies on certain individual or group activities and practices in order to be sustained and expressed.' This view resonates with Wilcock's (1999) vision of spirituality in occupational therapy, which suggests that therapists can facilitate wellbeing for others by facilitating opportunities to participate in activities that are best fitted to their personality and wishes and reflect who they want to become. This means that in terms of life balance, spirituality is closely associated with an individual's sense of *fulfillment* and with having sufficient time and energy for involvement in a *variety* of different life activities, at least some of which are *meaningful* as well as *productive* or *purposive*. We touched on these words previously, but I want to revisit them here to clarify why they are important in relation to spiritual wellbeing and a sense of personal identity.

MEANINGFUL AND PRODUCTIVE ACTIVITIES

As I have mentioned previously, activities that are *personally meaningful* are the things that you enjoy doing because they give you a personal sense of fulfillment, pleasure or joy. Often, these kinds of activities are *identity affirming* because they represent an aspect of who you are or who you would like to be or become. Meaningful activities can also be purposive, but in affluent Western economies, these types of activities are frequently associated with usefulness or productivity and have a sense of symbolic capital or value to those societies.

As members of these social environments we have become acculturated to the need to be both *useful* and *productive* if we are to be considered of value to significant others and our wider society. Whilst this is very important to our sense of belonging and community, sadly productivity is frequently used synonymously with *paid work*. This is unfortunate because many types of daily activities are productive (or purposive) in one way or another, not least the unpaid realms of domestic labor, or the altruistic voluntary and community spirit underpinning citizenship or social responsibilities.

By ignoring these 'other' kinds of productive activities and associating value and usefulness exclusively with paid labor, so we exclude the more egalitarian aspects of caring and community networks. As noted previously, this kind of practice is ethically unsound and belies the caring and relational aspects of life as well as the value of meaningful occupation to achieve wellbeing as opposed to the ever-increasing demands from paid work:

> The employment agenda should not be ruled by the dictate of business needs but by human needs such as rest, leisure, caring for dependents, the welfare of children and giving people the opportunity to meet their full human worth; the economy should be the servant of our needs not our master. (Bunting 2005, p.xxvii)

WHAT IS A SENSE OF SELF OR SELF-IDENTITY?

There are several different theories about what constitutes a self-identity, but most suggest three key elements are required. These are having a sense of *biographical continuity* or *sameness* through time (e.g. as one progresses through the life cycle); a sense of coherence or *'ecological consistency'* (Grote and Raeder 2009, p.222) in one's behavior within and across different life domains such as paid work, home, community, social and leisure pursuits; and third, a personal sense of autonomy or self-determination over life events and activities, and therefore some element of an *internal locus of control* or self-determination (choice) about how you spend your time and energy.

As I have discussed earlier, occupational therapists not only emphasize the need for choice, but also emphasize the importance of participation in personally meaningful activities as a predominant and required factor to find meaning and purpose in life.

Wilcock (1999) began the process of sketching a theory of occupation that would be dependent upon meaning rather than specifically upon purpose. She observed that while some theorists see daily life as comprised of goal-directed, purposeful activities, it is, in fact, much more than just 'doing' things but rather a synthesis (or dynamic balance) of *doing, being* and *becoming* types of activities:

> A dynamic balance between doing and being is central to healthy living and wellness… Doing… is so important it is impossible to envisage the world of humans without it. Being encapsulates such notions as nature and essence, about being true to ourselves, to our

individual capacities and in all that we do. Becoming adds to the idea of being a sense of future and holds notions of transformation and self-actualization. (Wilcock 1999, p.1)

This approach to balance is common in occupational science and therapy and has two clear aspects: first, life is multifaceted and multidimensional so balance must take consideration of this complexity; and second, that the meaning of life is important to wellbeing. However, I would suggest that life would have to have a *meaning orientation* and not a *performance* one if this kind of model and belief were to be realized.

DOING, BEING, BECOMING AND BELONGING ACTIVITIES

If life balance is about being focused on meaning and not performance, then it is about how you personally feel about an activity and not just its purpose, especially as measured in terms of socially expected obligations. Western cultures are predicated on a model of doing, creating not only a performance orientation in paid work but general busyness in life. Consequently, if we apply Wilcock's (1999) theory of finding life balance through a synthesis of active 'doing' activities, reflexive 'being' and 'becoming' pursuits as a means of achieving a state of balance and wellbeing in everyday life, then we have to challenge this hegemony of a doing and performance orientation to achieve a more integrated meaning-oriented perspective.

Other occupational scientists, such as Rebeiro *et al.* (2001) and Hammell (2011; 2004), have also illustrated the importance of adding a sense of belonging to Wilcock's notion of life balance, to capture the relational context and sense of place that exists in everyday relationships, networks and connections. For me this is an essential addition because every activity, every sense of 'being' in the world is held within a relational context as we are all socially and ecologically interconnected.

DOING

The concept of doing includes purposeful, goal-oriented activities and it is the basic action of everyday social interaction and societal growth (Wilcock 1999). It is 'doing' that is associated with paid and unpaid work because it is an active, purposive occupation.

Doing activities can be meaningful and research has identified five different ways people experience meaning through 'doing' including the opportunity to keep busy; to have something to get out of bed for (a purpose to the day); to explore new opportunities and to envisage a future in which *there is* time and energy to engage in personally valued activities; and to contribute meaningfully to others in the family, community and wider society (Hammell 2004).

The trouble is that 'doing' work, paid or unpaid, is the ultimate occupation in most societies who engage in the global market place and 'doing' has become fraught with pressures to do more to keep afloat in this competitive, profit-driven playing field. Consequently, people have speeded up to meet more and more demands and expectations on their use of time and energy. Many become exhausted or disenfranchized; others become plagued by the need to do too much and become addicted to that. I have already mentioned Hochschild's (2000) notion of busyness as the opiate of the masses but Schaef (2004, p.22) has broken this down, identifying not only the 'workaholic', who exclusively works, but also the 'rushaholic', the 'busyaholic' and the 'careaholic', all of whom 'do' to the exclusion of anything else.

These kinds of obsessive or excessive foci destroy any sense of meaning in life and bring me back to the crux of the problem; in many Western cultures we 'do' too much in paid and/or unpaid obligatory and/or purposive activities to the *exclusion of other types of activities,* and this is a bludgeoning problem, causing imbalance and ill-health because people are multidimensional and need to engage in other pursuits to facilitate growth and a meaningful sense of self in *all* dimensions of life.

BEING

Being has been defined as time taken to reflect, to be introspective or meditative, to (re)discover the self, to be aware of and live in the moment, to appreciate art or music, to enjoy being with those you care about or want to spend time with and very importantly, but often forgotten in our busy lives, to value and spend time with nature in a contemplative and appreciative manner (Hammell 2004).

These kinds of activities (or *occupations*, i.e. all the things we do every day) tend be activities we find personally meaningful because, quite simply, we get pleasure from spending time in them or find them restorative and health giving because we need reflective time, contemplation and creative expression; they balance our busyness and our active doing and allow us to replenish energy levels:

> To live as a fully self-actualizing person involves the process of being, of simply experiencing life and the environment around us, frequently in an accepting, non-instrumental way. Being, in this sense, involves the realms of meaning, value, and intentionality that imbue our lives with a richness and diversity that transcends what we know and what we do. (Rowles 1991, p.265)

Being activities are not necessarily defined as socially purposeful, which *doing* activities frequently are, because they are not actively linked to paid work. This means they tend to exist outside of the expected or socially defined *obligatory* things we have to do every day and consequently are *freely* and *actively* chosen by the individual rather than socially scripted. Maslow (1968, p.233) describes 'being' as the 'contemplation and enjoyment of the inner life... antithetical to action in the world i.e. it produces stillness and cessation of muscular activity'. For Maslow (1968), experiencing a state of 'being' is necessary to achieve self-actualization and the peak experience of life, a state of flow, 'in which time disappears and hopes are fulfilled' (p.233). Self-actualized people experience the world more holistically, more richly and with a greater sense of belonging than those who never reach this level of experience. These people:

> Appreciate again and again, freshly and naively, the basic goods of life, with awe, pleasure, wonder and even ecstasy, however stale those experiences may have become to others. Thus, for such a person any sunset may be as beautiful as the first one, any flower may be of breath-taking loveliness, even after he has seen a million flowers...For such people, even the casual workaday, moment-by-moment business of living can be thrilling, exciting and ecstatic (Maslow 1954, pp.214–215).

Consequently, the term 'being' is also used to describe our personal sense of self: being present in and a part of our everyday world; *how* we are (behave, feel, respond) in the world. This touches on our self-identity and having an awareness of *who we are* and *what we want* and value in life and is part of the journey toward becoming self-actualized. Grote and Raeder (2009, pp.222–223) have described the importance of 'biographical continuity' (a continual sense of the same self across time), 'ecological consistency' (having a personal sense of coherence in one's behavior across different domains of life) and 'locus of control' in terms of its internal or external relevance necessary to forming and building on one's self-identity over time. This is reflective of Carl Rogers' (1961) notion of finding congruence between who you want to be and who you actually are and, of course, who you *can* actually become.

BECOMING

Becoming describes the idea that people can envision possible future selves and potentialities, achieve ideas about who and what they might want to become over time or through their lifespan, and attain a personal sense of congruence between who they want to be and who they do actually become.

According to Fidler (1983), there are three facets to becoming: these are becoming 'I' (an integrated sense of self-identity); becoming competent (achieving personal mastery or self-determination); and becoming a social being (achieving congruence with self and others and a sense of relationships with others). These link back to the ideas of ecological consistency, biographical continuity and locus of control in terms of developing a self-identity: becoming is about being true to yourself, and, significant to Roger's (1961) theories, achieving congruence between the 'ought' self (what I should do/be/become), the ideal self (what I want to do/be/become) and the real or actual self (what I actually do/am/am becoming), so is a process of self-actualization. Becoming, then holds the notion of achieving personal growth and potential, of transformation and self-actualization.

BELONGING

Belonging needs are about relationships, which can vary across a broad spectrum, from everyday social interactions to more significant friendships, thus can encompass daily happenstances, workplace associations, social support networks and familial love and caring relationships. These kinds of social and personal encounters tend to be reciprocal, which means they meet our mutual needs for being cared for, loved, liked, or valued by and meaningful to others. Belonging is also about having a *sense of place*, somewhere to settle, to be a part of and feel safe or secure in.

Of course the problem with achieving a sense of belonging, like all of the dimensions, is that in neoliberalism, it can be challenged. Individualism is promoted over collectivism or connectivity, i.e. a sense of belonging and community and even to some extent family, because paid work can be divisive in forming and maintaining relationships. Yet, understanding connections, not only between people, but between the myriad life activities and the basic contours of daily life, is the way to go forward.

Caproni (2004) argues that notions of work–life balance are viewed too strategically, disregarding complexity and that 'life is, and probably should be, deeply emotional, haphazard, and uncontrollable' (Caproni 2004, p.213). I agree and purport that balance is, in essence, living and breathing doing, being, becoming and belonging activities in an interconnected and meaningful way in our everyday lives.

CONCLUSION

To summarize then, life is complex and multidimensional, composed of an interrelated dance of doing, being, belonging and becoming activities. Yet, the neoliberal notions of work–life balance in Western economies are skewed by the constructs and value systems surrounding paid work. These constrain how the complex activities and interconnections of life necessary for wellbeing are perceived and understood: life has become two-dimensional, with paid work diametrically opposed to the rest of life, which in itself has become condensed into the home and caring domain. If you do only one or the other, then you will fill that up to the top with constant busyness. There is little or no place for a sense of being in the world, for contemplation and rest, for love and belonging or mutually supportive social connections; there is no time to become a self other than a worker, because this is not worthy of value and has no social capital.

So what if we challenged this and changed it? What kind of life balance would we have if it was born of connections and not control, of wellbeing and not productivity, of attention and not intensification, of meaning and not performance, of reconciliation and not compromise? After all, 'It is how we choose what we do and how we approach [life balance] that will determine whether the sum of our days adds up to a formless blur or to something resembling a work of art' (Csikszentmihalyi 1997, p.13) and I, for one, want my life to be beautiful.

CHAPTER 2
DOING TOO MUCH IN PAID WORK

INTRODUCTION

In this chapter I will discuss why people can do too much in paid work and how in Western economies we see paid work as a valued and significant *'doing'* activity, intricately linked with our personal identity, self-esteem and wellbeing.

Yet, whilst paid work holds this respected position in our society, we can also find that labor markets can be very greedy in terms of the amount of personal time and energy they take up (Coser 1974). *Intensification,* or in Paton's words (2001, p.63) 'do more with less culture' in terms of increased workloads, work pressures and expectations, has become endemic in our paid work environments and consequently, workers experience pressure and stress, causing not only dissatisfaction and ill-health, but significant life *imbalance.*

Unsurprisingly, because time and energy is over spent in the contract of paid work, other obligatory doing activities (like domestic chores, caring and family commitments) and the activities necessary for survival (like eating and sleeping), become the second level of priority outside of paid work, which leaves no surplus time and energy to do other types of activities or the things that may be personally meaningful or enjoyable, whether in fact these are doing, being, becoming or belonging types of activities.

Under these circumstance it is perhaps surprising that many people seem to consciously choose to prioritize paid work, even though this causes pressures to spill over into other life domains and creates a feeling of busyness in everyday life. But when we recognize that an overwork culture is the norm in the modern labor market, then we begin to see how shaped we are by our social structures, in this case the model of productivity, profit and consumerism purported by neoliberal capitalism. As Lefebvre (2004, p.74) puts it in this kind of model, 'There is not time to do everything but every "doing" has its time. These fragments form a hierarchy, but work remains to a large extent essential... the reference to which we try to refer everything else back.' These kinds of work-driven cultures create an interesting conundrum in our modern lives and underpin why *work–life imbalance*, and consequently imbalance in the whole of life, has become an insidious problem in Western economies.

Please note that in this and ensuing chapters I will be using stories and direct quotes from people working in the United Kingdom (UK) health and social care public services sector to give real life examples of these influences and I think their experiences will resonate with many of you who are reading this book, whether or not you work in such settings.

WHY ARE WE CREATING IMBALANCE BETWEEN PAID WORK AND LIFE?

People have to expend time and use energy to participate in daily activities, whether these are the active doing, the belonging, becoming or more reflective, being pursuits. As we engage in our daily lives we weave across multiple life domains, and whilst a balance between these different types of activity is necessitated for a personal sense of coherence and wellbeing in life, because of how we have structured our everyday lives in Western economies, we tend to prioritize the domains of paid work and then other obligatory activities, such as home or caring commitments.

Indeed, for most people these two activities take up most of our daily rations of time and energy and if one domain (usually paid work) is greedy and takes too much, then it depletes the reserves in the other. Hochschild (2000) has called the resulting sense of conflict and stress that people can experience through this practice of trying to balance these two domains the 'time bind'.

The problem with this rather exclusive emphasis on paid work and home or family responsibilities in Western economies is that it focuses solely on 'doing' the so-called paid, purposive and then unpaid obligatory tasks in life and overlooks the significance of spending time and energy in the not so valued, and consequently *non-obligatory* or *recreational* types of pursuits (Ransome 2008). This, in essence, excludes not only other 'doing' activities, but the being, belonging and becoming occupations. These other activities, outside of paid work and home domains, are socially classified as non-essential activities because the time and energy used to participate in them is not considered useful in a productive or economically profitable sense. The result is that these get squeezed into any personal time or energy reserves that are left over after paid work and unpaid home responsibilities are done, or are lost completely. As one occupational therapist described it:

> I would like to think that I was able to manage my workload in a contained time. Within, you know, 'work hard, play hard'. I don't think that's a bad philosophy really. But I think [paid work] does overlap because, even at the most basic level you're tired when you come home. And then you've got the responsibilities [unpaid home-based obligatory tasks]: the boring things like being a domestic goddess [laugh] like the cooking and then ironing and all that nonsense becomes a really big chore…

It would seem then, that work–life *im*balance is a product of the very social structures and workplace cultures that we as a society have created; it follows that where social norms describe this as the way to be in everyday life, so we, as subjects of that society, will strive to achieve it. Conversely, if we accept that it is participation in all activities, whether socially classified as obligatory or non-obligatory, that gives us meaning in everyday life, and that this promotes a coherent sense of self and wellbeing in life, then we *have to* find the time and energy reserves to participate in them if we are to live balanced lifestyles.

This of course leads us to the essence of the life balance problem: it is having the very space, time and energy reserves to expend in this way that is lacking in present life balance models *because* we focus on productivity and consumerism, often to the exclusion of everything else. Consequently, it is this mindset about life balance that we have to address because it is the variety, breadth and interconnected synergy of all daily activities in both the social and natural world that makes life worth living. As Gorz puts it, we should all be striving to participate in activities that are

> unrelated to any economic goal which are an end in themselves: communication, giving, creating and aesthetic enjoyment, the

production and reproduction of life, tenderness, the realization of physical, sensuous and intellectual capacities, the creation of non-commodity use-values (shared goods or services) that could not be produced as commodities because of their unprofitability – in short, the whole range of activities that make up the fabric of existence and therefore occupy a primordial rather than a subordinate place. (1980, pp.80–81)

WHY HAS WORK–LIFE IMBALANCE BECOME SO PROBLEMATIC?

In many ways we have already answered this question, but here I will revisit some of these points, as well as discussing some other key changes that have occurred which have made this problem more apparent.

As we know from earlier discussions, work–life balance is a term used to describe an ideological separation or division between paid work and the rest of life's activities, especially those activities associated with caring and the home. We also know that the challenge to find balance between paid work and home has become worse because of neoliberal capitalism which, by its direct action, drives a *performance orientation* and *intensification,* which pushes people to overwork. However, this problem has also been expounded by other social and demographic changes.

First, women, as the traditional carers and unpaid domestic workers, have moved into the paid labor market. This has served to directly juxtapose the two life domains of paid work and the home in a direct way. However, although the role of women as paid employees has expanded, the stereotypical expectations of them in the home have not decreased at the same rate (Gershuny, Bittman and Brice 1997; Gershuny, Godwin and Jones 1994). This means that working women and their employing organizations have had to accommodate greater conflict scenarios between paid work and home than ever before, and the notion of workers, specifically women, having to juggle both work and home commitments, was born.

Second, political drivers have promoted an adult labor model, which expects all people of working age, irrespective of caring commitments, personal challenges or choices to participate in paid work. This means single parents, carers, people who have specific requirements or disabilities, and those who are unemployed or retired are encouraged to participate in the paid work arena in some way; but, and this is a big problem, little, if anything, is done to support them and this facilitates conflict and imbalance.

Third, people are living longer and consequently requiring the support of families for lengthier periods of time. This is increasing the caring commitments of working adults, leading to the emergence of the so called 'sandwich generation,' who support both children and older relatives (Greenhaus 2008, p.343).

These kinds of changes have begun to influence how we think about the traditional gendered divisions of labor and consequently have begun to emphasize the importance of achieving and maintaining life balance for men as well as women:

It has challenged and restructured the old institutions of production, reproduction and the state in ways that have radically transformed relations of dependence and care between people and social groups and the assumptions about gendered responsibility that held these spheres [of paid work and life] together. (McDowell 2004, p.146)

THE WORKPLACE, FAMILY AND WIDER NETWORKS

Neoliberal work regimes are, according to Capra (1996, p.11), 'life destroying' and 'life draining' and yet this pattern of work continues, with impunity, in modern labor markets.

When we consider that our workplaces are human organizations, living communities of people who are in relationships with significant others, not only in the workplace, but outside of it, the key question to ask must be why do we continue to take too much of the individual's time and energy reserves into paid work? We know that this practice will not only influence the individual worker's health and wellbeing, but will also impact on the quality of their relationships with families and their social and community networks, as well as the relational ties they have with significant others within the fabric of the workplace itself. Think about it; if you are exhausted and busy all the time, you have little time to invest in the quality of your relationships with others, even if they share the same office space. Consequently, the sense of belonging and therefore commitment that you have, both with the organization you work in and the individuals who make up that network, is challenged.

By the very nature of our interconnections of self with others and both our social and natural worlds beyond paid work, these kinds of pressures also impact on our participation in and relationship with our social and community domains, as well as the far less considered, but perhaps even more important, natural environment from which we are alienated, because there is no time and energy left to appreciate it.

This kind of practice can result in several dilemmas for working people and their networks (families and co-workers), which I am going to describe here using the stories of those real people I told you about previously – in this case occupational therapists working in health and social care organizations in the UK. Both these settings are large, bureaucratic, public sector (state funded) organizations, but the stories shared will resonate for many us who work in very different workplaces.

THE SEVEN DILEMMAS OF WORK–LIFE IMBALANCE
THE DILEMMA OF INTENSIFICATION AND STRESS

In both the organizations accessed, the occupational therapists that participated in the study described how the pressures in paid work appeared to be intensifying and that this was an on-going problem:

> You know, maybe it's rose tinted glasses, but I'm sure I can remember a time when you had peaks and troughs... You'd have really busy periods and then you'd have quieter periods. And that just doesn't happen anymore. It's like it's relentless.

As noted previously, intensification is a problem in neoliberal capitalism. The drive to make profit, be competitive and/or productive means that workers are expected to do more work in less time, driving a performance orientation and causing pressure to work longer and longer hours in order to get the expectations of the job done; this breeds a pervasive culture of overwork.

Stories of multitasking were rife, with the working day described as being like 'a constant juggling act' or 'like spinning plates... rushing from one to the other to keep things going.' In all reported cases this created a sense of stress, because paid work was seeping into people's personal lives, taking time and energy away from other activities in a physical, psychological and emotional sense. Commonly reported as leading to stress and ill-health, descriptions of 'sleepless nights mulling things over' and other associated psychological and emotional disturbances were endemic, recounted even by those who identified work as a something they enjoyed:

And I don't mind working hard. And I don't mind giving the hours. It's when it impacts on other things and I feel I'm not being able to cope with it. That's when I get stressed. Because I think I'm not actually coping with this. And when you wake up at sort of 3 o'clock in the morning and you're planning out treatment plans for people, that's the time you know it's really getting to a point where it's a bit of an overload.

These stories were accompanied by beliefs that these increasing pressures were either unrecognized, ignored or, frankly, unsupported in the workplace, even though it was blatantly apparent that more and more was expected in a day's work, draining individual reserves: 'You know the more you're prepared to give, the more the kind of system will suck out of you basically.' This was accompanied by a sense that you had to physically speed up to achieve what you needed to get done, as more and more was expected in the working day, increasing pressure and stress:

But the danger is that you keep taking on, taking on. And then eventually, you know, you feel like a hamster on a wheel. And you think, stop! I need to get off. Because the faster you run, the faster the wheel goes, and the faster you have to go to keep on it.

Interestingly, although participants identified the pressures of paid work as causal to their sense of stress and imbalance, a second emergent theme was a perception of having very little, if any, personal autonomy over this, and consequently a reported inability to change these pressures in the workplace in any meaningful way.

THE DILEMMA OF A LACK OF CONTROL AND CHOICE

There was a strong sense that externalized organizational drivers – pressures to discharge people in the health settings and to reduce waiting lists in the social care setting – were creating immense work-based stresses and that little could be done by individual respondents to address it. Rehabilitation services, for example, were given a 'ten day snapshot' and consequently 'to get things sorted out you're going some.' Similarly, working on acute medical wards meant 'a 48 hours stay. You've got to work within that context... within those confines, really.'

Others railed that they had no control or decision-making power (personal autonomy or self-determination) over workload management or time spent in the workplace because externalized pressures directed this, causing their levels of stress to rise exponentially: 'But that puts horrendous pressure on. And I've been known to be here until 9 o'clock at night just finishing data, which is wanted for the next morning.'

A lack of control over working time and load has been commonly noted as a product of neoliberal labor principles and highlighted as a causal factor in work–life imbalance. After all, if you have no personal sense of personal autonomy, self-determination or an *internal locus of control* over your own workloads and working hours because others hold this power, then you cannot *freely* choose when and how you work.

Control is a difficult word in the personal context because it holds connotations of power and coercion and from that perspective can be quite negative. However, this is a notable point in terms of work–life balance, because when power over the individual is perceived as held by others, i.e. an *external locus of control*, then you, as that individual, feel you have no personal autonomy or choice over your own decisions about work–life balance. Alternatively, an *internal locus of control* purports a *personal sense of autonomy* or *self-determination* over your own work–life balance. Consequently, this is something we should strive for.

In the stories shared here the *control*, that is, decision-making and choice over work–life balance was experienced as held by more powerful others, that is, an *external locus of control*. This externalized sense of power is a real problem in the neoliberal workplace because labor markets have to be managed in order to be effective, make profit and be competitive or productive; if people are the resource required to achieve this, then they become a tool to be used, to best advantage, in the cycles of production. Consequently, neoliberal markets are very powerful tools in controlling the worker and pushing performance indicators, creating that performance orientation in all of us and eroding a personal sense autonomy and self-determination. As Coyle succinctly puts it, in the neoliberal workplace:

> New inequalities of time are manifest: between those who have some power to bargain over the definition of working time and those do not; between those who are able and willing to comply with the requirements to extend their working time and those who are not; and those who can resist flexibilization and intensification and those who cannot. (2005, p.88)

This sense of limited power was very notable in the stories shared, but the most insidious element of this spiraling sense of limited control was that participants felt they had little or no ability to challenge it, because of a pervasive sense of fear about repercussions in the workplace should they do so. In essence, this meant that the occupational therapists felt compelled or coerced to meet organizational demands, however great these were and despite their leading to endemic life imbalance, because they feared there would be consequences if they did not comply.

THE DILEMMA OF A CULTURE OF FEAR AND INSECURITY

Occupational therapists in both settings commented that they felt all employees invariably conceded to organizational demands, however greedy or excessive they were, because they feared potential repercussions, for example having their 'card marked for later on.' They used the euphemism of a 'culture of fear' to capture this sense of insecurity:

> It's almost as if there's a kind of culture of fear in work–life balance really. And I won't, kind of, dare step out of line for fear of the consequences. And, you know, possibly with some justification. Because there's always this kind of implied threat hanging over people. If you step out of line you may not lose your job, but life can be made difficult for you. And your promotion prospects might diminish.

To feel threatened or coerced into working longer and harder because you actually feel this will be detrimental to your career is a terrible indictment of contemporary working practices, and this sense of fear was rife.

It is an interesting dichotomy of neoliberal discourse that the drive for individualism, i.e. putting the rights of the individual before the group and purporting that you, as an individual, can live your life as you choose to in terms of achieving personal goals, personal uniqueness and personal autonomy, has actually resulted in *less choice* and *greater scrutiny* and *control* over the working person in terms of life balance. This offers a cautionary tale, identifying how the apparent movement of power from the state to the individual citizen can, in fact, be no more than rhetoric because, in practice, the power is actually consolidated within the edifice (state or organization). This is blatantly apparent in terms of work–life balance, where the process of flexibilization, namely, increased patterns of flexible working in the labor market, has in fact *limited* the autonomy of the individual employee and *increased* the power and control that organizations hold over this. Fundamentally, this means that traditional patterns of work become more flexible, but you are subject to the whim of others in terms of when and how you work, and this can cause conflict (here we go again) with your commitments outside of work:

> Employers are freer to schedule work across evenings and weekends and employees need to be available to work during those times. Not only has working time become flexible, but so has non-work time, which can no longer be planned on a fixed or permanent basis. (Coyle 2005, p.80)

Strangely enough, it was very clear in the stories shared that a little more give, as opposed to take, on behalf of the managers in the organizations could have substantially reduced conflict between paid work and life in meaningful ways for employees, without, one could assume, damaging or long-term effects on organizational outcomes; and yet, this was not implemented. It seems a simple question to ask these organizations and their incumbent managers why they did not try a little harder to meet personal requirements in terms of flexible working for staff if it could have improved the employee's experience. The answer, unsurprisingly, always came back to the same thing: limited money and resource constraints.

THE DILEMMA OF RESOURCE CONSTRAINTS

Several respondents who were managers in their respective settings reported that they felt constrained by organizational priorities and barriers such as resource implications in the application of flexible working policies. It seemed managers identified constraints in how they would like to give employees greater choice over when and how they worked to support work–life balance but felt they could not, in fact, do this because, as a matter of course, the individual's choices in terms of patterns of work had to be measured against the impact it would have on the organization's performance indicators; and this was inevitably found wanting:

> We have looked for one girl for compressed hours because she's got home commitments. So there are sort of opportunities out there. I think the difficulty comes then, in whether or not you can argue your case sufficiently against your service needs. [See Box 2.1a,b for more examples]

These structural limitations made it difficult for managers to instigate work–life balance policies fairly, even though policies were in place, because occupational therapy staff *were* the resource to deliver the service effectively (see Box 2.1c). As a result of this approach opportunities for staff were experienced as limited, and there was a sense that work–life balance opportunities were inequitable:

> But I can remember it being said right at the outset. It's gonna be, to a certain extent, a kind of first-come-first-served type business. Because inevitably there would be a kind of cap, if you like, on the number of people who are able to work flexibly. So that's a difficult one. Because that, in a sense, is inherently unfair.

Box 2.1 The dilemma of resource constraints over employee work–life balance

a. 'There's flexi-leave and then there's working compressed hours. You can also do working from home. These are all strategies that are endorsed by the organization. It's just finding the time and the resources to meet everybody's needs. Not everybody can do this.'

b. 'You would like to facilitate a work–life balance. It's something that I support. But service demands are sometimes so great that you can't facilitate it. I mean, we have a go down the year, but it's not always achievable for the individual.'

c. 'There isn't much room for error. And that's where it's difficult for the individual to carry out work–life balance in reality. And that's what it is in [the organization]. Rhetoric. And that's the difference between the rhetoric and the reality of work-life balance.'

THE DILEMMA OF EMOTIONAL SUPPORT AND CARE

What happens when organizations place money and resources before staff wellbeing and are perceived to be unequal in how they divvy up opportunities for support? Well unsurprisingly both organizations were considered to be inadequate in their provision of practical and emotional support for their employees. In particular there was little evidence of support for the emotional context of care, 'the need to provide attention, stimulation and love' for others (Holt and Thaulow 1996, p.84).

Occupational therapists told painful stories of not being able to take time off to care for children when they were sick; of being kept on at work when they should be picking their children up from school or childminders; of being refused compassionate leave for a funeral when there was a death in the family, and of exclusion from promotion, because as a carer for a very sick relative, someone could not work full-time.

Of course formal policies to support all these personal dilemmas existed in all the organizations; but their implementation was constrained not only by limited resources and the focus on organizational outcomes, but also by the normative acceptance that this was OK in the values of the organizational cultures, and this was interesting. I suppose the first thing you have to ask yourself in this situation is, why would profit or production be placed before people? Surely in a democratic, egalitarian and morally principled culture, social policies should be based not on the obligation to work to the exclusion of caring for others and indeed for yourself, but on the notion of reciprocal support to sustain the relationships of nurturing and caring for people by others; a relational network of caregiving if you like:

> A democratic ethic of care starts from the idea that everybody needs care and is (in principle at least) capable of care giving, and that a democratic society should enable its members to give both these activities a meaningful place in their lives if they so want. (Sevenhuijsen 2000, p.15)

It is this need for a caring perspective that resonated with the experiences shared by the occupational therapists. Participants described how they *wanted* to care for others, but were constrained in terms of achieving a work–life balance because of the limitations and expectations of the workplace and its culture, and described how this caused genuine and heartfelt ethical and moral dilemmas. Amber, for example, sent her young child to school when she was ill because she could not get carer's leave:

> I thought she'd [daughter] probably gone past the worst of it. But she's actually just got over tonsillitis and a respiratory tract infection. That's been two weeks. Now she's got conjunctivitis. And you think... I mean she's gone to school because they don't treat conjunctivitis anyways. They can't do anything for it. And she's only got it because she got it from her best friend [laugh]. But it's, you know... Well there's going to be things that she's still going to get. Hopefully it [child being sick] won't be too bad.

This may seem blithe, but the outcome for Amber (let alone her young child) was traumatic and the guilt she felt as a mother was palpable. Carer's leave was available in the organization, but it was only in an emergency situation. In terms of a child being sick, this meant it was only applicable on the first day of illness, then you needed to find other support systems. Now of course this is fair, isn't it? If you have a child and choose to work, that is your problem, isn't it? And of course, if you have to work, because you need the money, but you cannot manage the child-care commitments, then that is your problem too and perhaps, if it is challenging, you should not have had children.

Well yes, you can use any of those arguments, but when even using your own annual leave or taking unpaid leave is not available because others are unavailable to cover your work, as Amber intimated, you do have to wonder if the organization could have been just a little bit forthcoming, especially when you consider this is a workplace that employs predominantly women. Also, do remember that Amber (as a mother) was far from alone in her dilemma. Others talked about pressures to change working patterns (see Box 2.2a) or refusals to attend funerals (Box 2.2b), so it was not just caring that was problematic; it was flexibility.

> **Box 2.2 Ethical and moral dilemmas and upset**
>
> a. 'They [healthcare] actually asked me to change my days because I worked on Tuesday, Wednesday and Thursday and they needed me to work on Monday… And I mean it wasn't a requirement of the job, it was just a request. But they [healthcare] brought it up quite a lot. Even though I said it would be difficult, it was still brought up quite a lot so I did manage to do it. But it was quite difficult because I did have to change my childminder because my childminder couldn't work on a Monday. And she couldn't work Friday. Which is why I had chosen [to work on] Tuesday, Wednesday and Thursday… So [childminder] lost her job. [Child] was upset and unsettled for weeks. And me. Well I was just mad. Seething. Still am. I just don't think that's fair.'
>
> b. 'I requested special leave. My Godfather died. So when he died it really just was so upsetting for me that I needed special leave off. When I asked for it, it was, "No you don't have special leave for things like that. No. Because he's not a close relative." Which I found really interesting; because for me it was really important'.

By structuring work as the ethically and morally 'right' activity to do and citing this as important, if not *more* important than caring and family commitments, so we have polarized two ethical elements of everyday life in the work–life balance continuum and created more than a compromise between two conflicting sets of values: 'family values: caring, sharing, non-competitive, focus on cohesion' and 'marketplace values: competitive rivalry, achievement orientation, individualism, excellence' (Hakim 2006, p.287), we have also created a lack of meaning, value and purpose in our relationships with both self and others, and placed all notions of self-worth and sense of purpose in life in one basket, that is, with the notion of participation in paid work and our interactions with the values of neoliberal capitalism. These kinds of pressure make paid work and the ability to achieve life balance for the employee even harder, and underpin the next dilemma, where the drives for greater performance reduce employee wellbeing and directly cause ill-health.

THE DILEMMA OF PERFORMANCE VERSUS HEALTH AND WELLBEING

Stories of ill-health and stress as a result of the pressures in paid work were prolific, citing physical load and psychological worries as casual factors:

> Even the four days I had off in between I would be thinking about work all that time. And by the Sunday I would be still be thinking about work. What have I got tomorrow? I never knew what I would go into, you know? So yes. It really affected me. I was ill. I lost a lot of weight. And I was sort of a person that didn't like taking time off sick, so I was going in whatever, you know?

The idea that there is a correlation between an increase in stress and pressures at work and a reduction in subjective wellbeing is well argued in the literature. Much of this is about the intensified sense of overwork we have in modern societies and the competing demands this creates between the time and energy needed in paid work and for home commitments, causing a frenetic dance of stress and imbalance:

> My waiting list used to be around three months. Now it's around a year… Daft isn't it when you think I'm here trying to work on people's stress levels. Never mind healer, heal thyself. What about healthcare caring for the health of the staff? That one's long gone.

A study by the Mental Health Foundation in 2003 specifically asked employees about their hours of work and their associated sense of wellbeing. A third of respondents ($n = 557$) felt unhappy or very unhappy about the time they devoted to work. More than 40 per cent of people reported neglecting other aspects of their life because of paid work and believed this increased their vulnerability to mental health problems. Twenty-seven per cent of people believed working long hours increased their levels of depression, whilst 34 per cent felt they were more anxious and 58 per cent more irritable and tense.

The study also highlighted that people felt longer hours at work increased the time they used to think or worry about work, and identified that as their weekly hours in work increased, so did their feelings of unhappiness. Women reported more unhappiness than men (42% of women compared with 29% of men), which was associated with higher levels of competing life roles and more pressure to 'juggle' paid work and life commitments. In essence, people were neglecting 'the factors in their lives which make them resistant or resilient to mental health problems' (Mental Health Foundation 2003, p.4), i.e. the loving and caring and the personally meaningful doing, being, belonging and becoming pursuits that exist in life outside of paid work.

Several other studies have identified that ill-health and stress are directly related to the drive to overwork in neoliberal capitalism (e.g. Brannen 2005; Costea, Crump and Amiridis 2008; Sennett 1998), creating the pressure to prioritize paid work over family, caring commitments and personal wellbeing. Gergen (2000, p.175) has identified how we have lost the capacity to sustain close and meaningful friendships because we are always 'in motion', constantly busy in some form of doing, and consequently have no time to invest meaningfully in each other. Social media as the communication channel of the new technological age comes to mind here; a great tool for sharing across the boundaries of time and space, but what about its relational meaning? Text, avatars and emails have no physical proximity, eye contact or genuine tone of voice.

At another critical level, Adam talks of how the demands of paid work (and I would add busyness), have alienated us from the natural cycles of time and thus the planet and rhythms of life, and identifies how this can erode wellbeing:

> The genesis of the industrial way of life has been accompanied by an effort to put on ever firmer footings the difference between human

culture and nature, mental activity and the physicality of being, artefactual time and the rhythmicity of the cosmos. (2003, p.60)

This identifies a critical relational issue in terms of life balance; as humans we have become separated from the planet and yet we are reliant on it for our wellbeing and survival. There are few large businesses, corporations or political forces that fight to be shepherds of the planet, or fundamentally care about the interconnected networks of which we are an integrated part, and on which we depend for survival. This is an absence we need to address and I will come back to this point in Chapter 9.

If this is not enough, whilst we continue to pile all our activity eggs into the one paid work basket, modern labor markets are creating instability in that very activity; paid work is becoming less secure, more fragmented, with short term contracts and flexible working practices proliferating. Focused on individual productivity and developing an increased sense of responsibility in the worker to manage their workloads and performance successfully, so the modern workplace ensures the workers carry the can (responsibility) for any intended and unintended consequences from decisions made and performance strategies implemented (Costea *et al.* 2008). This is a sad edict in terms of where our interests lie in the world of neoliberal capitalism and how demoralizing the outputs and outcomes of that are, and leads to the seventh dilemma of work–life imbalance in the modern workplace.

THE DILEMMA OF 'SELF-IDENTITY' AS VALUED 'WORKER'

A sense of value at work is an integral part of everyday satisfaction and is closely associated with self-identity. This, of course, is very important, as what we *do* in terms of paid work is a mark of success and is imbued with *symbolic capital*, which means it legitimately holds a significant amount of social value (Bourdieu 1989, p.17).

The problem with this value-based approach to paid work in the neoliberal labor market is that the characteristics of this type of capitalism have increased flexibility in the workplace and partnered this with the ideology of individualism, which assumes an employee will take responsibility for his or her own actions and performance in the workplace. Accompany this with *de-facto* reduced autonomy in terms of choice and control over working patterns and workload, increased scrutiny and performance management and a cruel sense of fear that coerces you to work harder, then you begin to worry more about your performance and achievements in paid work and feel compelled to be a 'worthy' employee, in order to maintain your self-esteem, self-worth and sense of security. You worry about your performance and work harder which makes *you* the responsible agent for your own actions and output in the workplace, and indeed in the rest of life, and that is just what the employing organization wants, because then it can abdicate its responsibility to do so. As Schumacher has eloquently pointed out:

> A person's work is undoubtedly one of the most decisive formative influences on his character and personality... [but] The question of what the work does to the worker is hardly ever asked, not to mention the question of whether the real task might be to adapt the work to the needs of the worker rather than to demand that the worker adapt himself to the needs of the work – which means, of course, primarily to the needs of the machine. (1979, p.5)

Others have also argued this point, all noting a social and global need to challenge the values we inherently hold and perpetuate in modern capitalism (e.g. Bunting 2005; Caproni 2004; Gambles *et al.* 2006). Caproni, in particular, identifies the value of meeting aesthetic needs if human wellbeing is to be realized and recalls Strati's (1992, p.568) vision of achieving a 'feeling of beauty' in life to illustrate what she feels is missing in contemporary work–life balance discourse. Potently, she recalls her own personal journey towards achieving work–life balance, which was marked by participation in meaningful activities beyond, but also inclusive of, paid work:

> To transcend this language [of work–life balance], I had to create for myself a new language that privileged tranquility over achievement, contribution over success, and choice over status. I gave up the notion that I should find passion in my work and instead looked to where I could make the greatest contribution for the most people and sought to keep passion in the home with my husband and children. Although I am not an advocate of finding passion in my work, I do believe work can be fun as well as productive.

What is interesting about Caproni's journey is that she is challenging herself and others to think differently about what is valuable in life, putting her own health and her family before her career and success at work.

I see no reason why this kind of change is not possible; but to achieve it requires quite a fundamental adjustment; we need to value other identities such as mother or father, caregiver, partner, lover, friend, family member, community participant, social actor or citizen and participate fully in these roles and identities as much as, if not more than, the role of the self as paid worker. It also requires us to accommodate and validate the space, time and energy required to value the reflective and aesthetic needs we have in life because these are not just pleasurable pastimes, but necessary for a meaningful sense of being alive, of being in the world. This entails primary changes across all levels of human consciousness and ways of being in both our social and natural worlds and that, reciprocally, requires not only major personal adaption but socio-cultural-political and organizational change, because the choices we make and the way we live is shaped by the contexts in which we are embedded (see Figure 2.1); and surely, we have now reached a point that necessitates change. After all 'Work... is a greatly overrated pastime, and a re-evaluation of... this critical position is long overdue' (Levitas 2001, p.451).

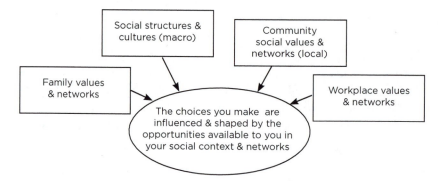

Figure 2.1 The complex web of influences acting on the choices you make

CONCLUSION

Many participants failed to make changes in how they were pressured to work, or to challenge inequity in policy application. Rather, they seemed to take for granted the way things were done in the organization on a daily basis, or adjust, under some duress, to make the most of the options they felt they had open to them. Participants were, as Hochschild (2000) has implicated in her own studies, *complicit* in the overuse of their own time and energy reserves in paid work; but this was because they were subject to the boundaries and control of work–life balance in the workplace, and accepted this as a taken-for-granted way of being in everyday life.

These patterns of being in the world are absorbed by people because significant others measure them as meaningful and purposeful and because social structures mirror them. I, for one, cannot say that this belief system is entirely wrong; paid work is an important component of life and gives meaning and identity to many and can be a personally meaningful activity, not just purposive, ideal or socially expected (Stebbins 2004).

However, although paid work can be both a productive and meaningful activity, because of the excessive demands of time and energy in paid work experienced by the occupational therapists in this study, many, even those who professed to love work, perceived very little sense of personal wellbeing in life. All were pressured or constrained in one way or another in achieving a meaningful work–life balance by the paid workplace. Conspicuous in its absence was not only diversity in everyday activities, but particularly, time to reflect, to think, or just to be present in life, with no evidence of time spent in the natural world at all. It is these lost or overlooked dimensions of time and activities that not only inhibit opportunities to reflect on how we are living our lives in the work-mad world of neoliberal capitalism and to challenge it successfully, but also prevents achieving a meaningful work–life balance and sustaining wellbeing.

CHAPTER 3
OBLIGATORY, NON-OBLIGATORY AND MEANINGFUL ACTIVITIES

INTRODUCTION

This chapter will discuss in more detail the impact of classifying caring commitments, domestic activities and paid work as the *obligatory* or *necessary* activities in modern life and other activities, however personally meaningful they are, as *non-obligatory* and consequently *unnecessary*, *less valued* and *less prioritized* in everyday life. I will describe why this is a very shortsighted view of life balance and how it actually *creates* and maintains over-busyness and imbalance in our everyday lives.

With examples, I will explore how this has become a specific concern for women workers, who at the moment predominantly, but not exclusively, carry the greatest load of unpaid domestic chores and caring commitments. However, I will also identify how the dance of over-obligation and over-busyness can be an issue for all people, irrespective of gender and, indeed, whether or not they are in paid employment.

OBLIGATIONS AND PAID WORK

However hard it might be to admit that this remains true today, in Western economies labor markets are sustained by models of paid work based on notions of the 'ideal type worker' (Callan 2007, p.674). In the traditional context, this was someone who worked in a full-time capacity, often in the same organization or line of work consistently over time, so had a career or 'job for life' and was fully committed to the workplace.

Now in the neoliberal labor market, this 'ideal' of the career-driven, usually male proponent of the breadwinner role has declined, morphing into the need for an ever more flexible individual, who, in essence, can work when required by the employing organization.

In this new world of flexibility in contracts and hours of work a 'just in time' (Odih 2003, p.293) approach to meeting organizational needs is becoming the norm. This means people are more and more frequently being employed just for when they are needed to do a particular job and have to be flexible in how they meet work time commitments (see Box 2.2a). Consequently, the 'ideal' worker is expected to develop a more portfolio or entrepreneurial approach to their career development. This is a far less stable working environment than the more traditional 'job for life' patterns of paid work, because workers may not be in either permanent or indeed full-time employment for any one organization at any one time or alternatively, they have to be ultra-flexible to meet workplace demands when required.

As mentioned previously, this kind of fragmented, temporal notion of flexibility can decrease the sense of security that we, as workers, have about paid work, and consequently can increase the feelings of worry and responsibility that we hold about our performance at work. However, because paid work and the rest of life are so intricately interconnected, we can also become more separated or decontextualized from both the home domain and all other activities outside of work that maintain our life balance, because time to work is so fragmented: 'The decoupling of work time from the time of the organization and from the collective rhythms of public and familial activities erodes communal activities in both the public and the private realm' (Adam 1995, p.103).

FLEXIBLE WORKING IN THE NEOLIBERAL WORKPLACE

Flexibility in paid work contracts has become a significant tool in neoliberal labor markets because flexible working patterns are viewed as effective, increasing the efficient use of resources and subsequently improving production and profit margins.

Of course if this is the outcome, then in a market economy based on competition, the method seems sound. However, the problem with this is that the resource being 'managed' in this effective way is human; it is people, and the outcome and wellbeing for the workers, their families and communities has not been so well considered, albeit the fact that flexible working is frequently cited as a valuable tool for enhancing work–life balance.

Now it cannot be denied that various forms of flexibility have been implemented and that these do offer opportunities for employees to work differently. These include:

- Temporal flexibility marked by flexibility in hours or patterns of work, e.g. the use of flexi-time and shift working.
- Locational flexibility defined as flexibility in the place of work, e.g. home working or hot desks in different work settings.
- Functional flexibility, which is changing or expanding job roles or job descriptions to accommodate different skill sets or practices.
- Financial flexibility emphasized through variable rates of pay, e.g. performance-related pay and bonuses.
- Numerical flexibility, or more open forms of employment like zero hour contracts, contract work or portfolio work (Grote and Raeder 2009, p.220).

On initial exploration these kinds of changes to the labor market may seem good. After all, if full-time work and the traditional idea of a 'job for life' is no longer significant, then people have greater freedom to work when they want to and Hakim's (2006) notion of greater choice in how we work, proposed in her preference theory (I discussed this in Chapter 1), becomes a viable reality to managing a good work–life balance.

However, and this is the nub of the problem, whilst some approaches to flexible working are not necessarily new (e.g. part-time working), the prominence of a 'just in time' approach to employment practices is. This has introduced a model of flexible working that is specifically marked by using *numerical* and *temporal* flexibility, both of which facilitate the process of matching staff resources to workplace demands as and when they are required. The problem with this kind of labor is that because it uses workers *when*, and indeed in some circumstances *if*, the organization needs them, then it dictates the hours and patterns of work, irrespective of how these collide with commitments outside of paid work.

Now this kind of practice can make you, as an employee, far more stressed as a consequence of trying to manage conflicts between work and home demands. Moreover, because of the neoliberal drive to make you, as a fully responsible adult, accountable for your actions in terms of managing those conflicts as well as your performance in the workplace, so you spiral into the moral and ethical dilemma of deciding if you place paid work before home, or home before paid work, neither of which is a real solution (remember Amber's experience mentioned in Chapter 2). By creating this conundrum for working people, so the traditional boundaries that existed between paid work time and non-work time in more fixed patterns of work break down, and this has consequences because, as discussed previously, this ultra flexible approach to paid work fragments time and changes the collective rhythms and patterns of family and community activities, so it creates greater work–life conflict.

Again, this impacts on working women because they frequently (but by no means exclusively) carry the greater load of responsibilities in the home domain, irrespective of the fact that they now participate in the paid work arena as commonly as men. People who carry these dual loads do have greater pressures to bear than those who have only one domain to consider, and this does lead to further problems in terms of meaningful participation in both paid work and home domains, whatever the individual's personal preferences may be in terms of priorities and choice. Let's look at some of these issues in more depth.

THE NEED FOR 'ZERO DRAG'

Perhaps one of the most worrying consequences of these new ways of flexible working is that employees not only have to show their commitment to the workplace through being very flexible (in order to be at work to meet work demands when they are needed), but also have to be *fully present* when they are in the workplace in order to assure that they are giving their full attention to the job in hand and are, consequently, value for money.

The problem with these kinds of expectations is that workers not only have to be ultra flexible to feel secure in the neoliberal workplace, they also have to evidence that they can be completely involved in their work 'at a full emotional level' (Coates 1997, p.1) in order to 're-create themselves as assets, to better the company' (Coates 1997, p.5). This of course can lead to the caring dilemmas I mentioned in Chapter 2 (how can I be at home for the kids/family when I have to do x, y and z at/for work?) and condones the issue of being responsible for your own decisions because you, as a fully responsible worker, carry the can for your own decisions about work and life, whatever the outcome, good or bad!

Hochschild (2000) has described the new type of 'ideal' worker as someone with 'zero drag' (p. xxiv): someone who is fully committed to their role as a paid worker without having any distractions to divert their attention from, or to conflict with, the time and energy needed for paid work.

In the neoliberal workplace, it is the singular and individualized approach to paid work and the fully committed attitude and performance orientation given to paid work, in whatever hours you work and in whatever job you do, that is the measure of success. It is this kind of approach that ensures the workplace has the best use of the human resource and has the value for money it craves, irrespective of the outcome on the worker and his or her family.

What are you thinking?

Now as you sit there and read this, just check what is going through your mind. You may think that this kind of approach to paid work is a good philosophy. After all, we *should* all work and it is this activity that means we can consume (buy stuff), as well as maintain productivity and growth of our economy and sustain the health and safety of our family; but what are the costs?

We know from the discussion in Chapter 2 that when paid work has this kind of philosophy embedded in its culture, it can affect your health and cause stress in family networks by reducing meaningful participation in these and indeed other non-paid life domains.

But what is also now clear is that there are other downsides: first, the philosophy of zero drag, of having no baggage or distractions to take your attention away from the workplace, *includes* children and other caring commitments; second, because the majority of carers are predominantly women, these practices can create bias in terms of achieving the status of the 'ideal' worker for women.

THE INTRANSIGENT CULTURE OF INEQUALITY

As mentioned earlier, neoliberal workplaces expect people to be ultra-flexible, that is, work whenever is needed and sustain a full-on commitment to work when in the workplace. This means, as workers, you have to maintain a flexible approach in response to workplace demands and be fully present in work when needed. Consequently, you need to have few, if any, distractions or responsibilities outside of paid work that take your time and attention, especially if those demands are time-specific, because this makes you less flexible than those workers who are not so tied (or have 'zero drag'), and consequently this means you are less profitable in the labor market.

Now women, of course, as the traditional purveyors of domestic, child and elder care commitments do tend to carry the greater load of responsibilities in the home domain. This means more women have to dance more frequently and more intensely with obligations in non-paid domestic roles as well as their paid work responsibilities, and because these kinds of responsibilities are frequently fixed or time-tied, they cannot be as flexible as men or women without these kinds of commitments.

This brings us back to the notion of individual choice in the flexible labor market: yes there are more opportunities to work flexibly in these markets *because* flexible patterns of work are becoming naturalized, BUT it only works for you (as the worker) if you can work when *you* need to around your fixed home commitments, and very few organizations work on that premise: they want you to be flexible enough to meet their needs.

THE PERFECT FIT

Now of course you can be lucky and you might just find the perfect fit in terms of your working time requirements and the organization's, but the rhetoric of having choice about when you work often outweighs the reality, and whilst you may not lose your job through your lack of flexibility, it may well impact on your prospects of promotion. Take for example the experience of Jenna, a part-time occupational therapist, who could not work full-time because she was caring for an ill relative:

> I've certainly compromised on promotion. And yes. That's where the compromise is. And part of me feels frustrated about that. But balanced with the way you knew what you were doing; that you knew that you'd have to take responsibility for that. But there is still part of you thinks, 'Well that's a bummer'. But that's how it actually had to be. How it is. And how it still is.

What is fascinating about Jenna's story is that she so clearly takes the responsibility for her choice and believes her decision was the right one, and of course she did *choose* to work part-time; but that choice was inevitable –

it was not a truly free choice, it was a moral, ethical and human one because to care for another is what we as human beings *should* do and *want* to do:

> These non-coerced *yet not voluntarily chosen* associations fill our lives. They range from the most intimate familial relations to those of fellow citizen and fellow traveller. Duties incurred by these associations arise out of a whole network of expectations, bonds, and responsibilities, most of whose validity we do not question, even if we question some specific obligations they impose. (Kittay 1999, p.62)

The policies to support Jenna's need to care and participate in paid work were there; indeed she was working part-time, but the culture to support her to progress developmentally, as a part-time worker, was not. She was categorically told that she would *have to* work full-time if she wanted to hold a more senior role, yet there was little to validate this cultural belief in the workplace other than its normative everyday practice.

So why was this a necessary requirement? Simply, the organization believed the position required a *full-time* and *full on* commitment and if Jenna rescinded her caring responsibilities, she would have zero drag and could apply for the position. What is sad about this is that Jenna was extremely experienced and skilled; she had the specific profile and qualification required for the role, and this particular profile was not easy to come by. Nonetheless, she was unrequited in her offer to work part-time in the position and was excluded from applying because she could not work full-time. For Jenna, this gave a very clear message: 'You're only a proper OT [occupational therapist] if you're a full-timer. So interesting. Yes. That's it, you know. And I know now that's sort of how it is.'

These kinds of compromises or trade-offs, which people make because of socio-cultural ideals, challenge the plausibility of Hakim's (2006; 2007) preference theory. If you recall from Chapter 1, this proposes that in the flexible labor market people have more options and make active choices to be either work-centered, family-centered or both (adaptive).

Now whilst I agree these options may be there, and that people can and do make these choices, they are constrained by the socially acceptable norms about paid work and caring in their social structures, workplaces and family networks and are significantly limited by the amount of responsibilities they carry as individuals.

Judging this as inequitable, Reiter (2007) has argued that in order to address this, organizations need to take a more ethical stance toward their models of flexibility and specifically promote a more person-centered or 'situationist' perspective in their application. This, she believes, facilitates optimum choice for the worker depending on his or her personal context, including their caring commitments, personal support systems, stakeholders, resources, and desires. She maintains that workplaces that do this will 'truly be employers of choice' (p.276) by sustaining the balance and wellbeing of employees and offering real options for those who cannot meet ideal expectations. I return to this issue of wellbeing in organizations in Chapter 8.

OBLIGATIONS IN LIFE

In the interim then, whilst we wait for organizations to catch up, what do we do to manage our obligations in life? Hochschild (2000, p.51) has illustrated that workers segment personal time and space into efficiency packets to manage their daily obligations effectively.

Identifying paid work as the 'first shift', the unpaid obligations and responsibilities at home as the 'second shift', and the emotional concerns, worries and guilt trips we hold about our responsibilities as family and community members as the 'third shift', Hochschild sees life as a rollercoaster of 'doing' obligatory things and feeling exhausted. Here I would like to look at some examples of this dance of the three shifts shared by occupational therapists from the study.

THE DANCE OF THE THREE SHIFTS

As well as the difficulties of managing her everyday commitments as a paid worker (shift 1), mother, wife and unpaid homeworker (shift 2), Maya, spoke of her commitments as a caregiver for older relatives as something she squashed into the weekends (shift 2). It was something she wanted to do, but it was beginning to feel challenging and that made her worry and feel guilty (shift 3):

> And I've got parents as well. I mean they're getting older and live up in XX. So I go there every Sunday. So that's again… They keep saying, 'Don't feel you have to come up.' But it's my time with them. And that's become a chore because that's the whole Sunday morning. And we're not back until after lunch. And then there's not much time to do anything in the afternoon. So that takes time out

as well. But I wouldn't have that any other way. I wouldn't want to not do that.

For Maya, the physical, emotional, psychological and ethical burdens were becoming heavy and she was conflicted about wanting to use her time to do this and feeling guilty that it used up more precious time and energy. She wanted more time with her children, time to cycle with her husband and 'me time' and it just was not there. Maya was not alone in her dance of the three shifts and the burden of guilt she carried.

Saffi, for example, was so busy with paid work and then family obligations that she had to manage her caring commitments for older adults by using her annual leave:

> And I think, you know, part of my problem is that a lot of my holidays are spent going back home. My father's quite disabled. So when I've got holidays, I feel I ought to go up there to support my mother because they don't have a carer. So it's like when you have got your holidays, a lot of the time it's going up there because I feel guilty that I should be going there.

The problem with both these stories, of course, is that the women are so busy doing the obligatory things in life that they feel they *have to do*, that there is no time or energy left for anything else. In both examples, they do *want* to care, but the time and energy constraints make it feel like a burden, and that makes them feel worse. This is a terrible dilemma yet is a common one because our life balance is so shaped by over-obligation and social expectations that we are constantly busy, and meaningful occupation, in terms of the things we do just for the sake of it, is lost. As Maya put it:

> It's getting the balance right between things you have to do and the things you enjoy doing. Which I am sure in this day and age is balanced more toward the things you have to do. 'I think we should be doing this.'

In the neoliberal context the 'shoulds' in life are obligatory activities: paid work is the ultimate goal with family roles and responsibilities a close second. Non-obligatory activities, which basically make up everything else in life, including community, leisure and social activities, as well as self-care, interests and personally meaningful activities, rank a poor third. In essence, all other types of doing outside of paid work and home/caring commitments, being, belonging and becoming types of pursuits are lost like chaff in the wind; this is ethically and spiritually crushing, leaving people feeling empty and wanting:

> Well I think [life] balance is about having a healthy balance between work, leisure and personal commitments. And I personally find that a struggle... But now I find that I'm sacrificing my personal time for my husband, my child, for work. And there's hardly any left at all for me. And so any sort of personal goals that I've got, you know, even if it's something simple like learning to speak Welsh or learning to ice skate, I just haven't got the time for. I just can't see me being able to fit in those leisure pursuits that I'd like to fit in. And I think it affects your self-esteem. It certainly affects my self-esteem. Because I just... I'm not a rounded person. I don't feel I'm a rounded person because I'm giving a lot of myself away to others really, I suppose, you know?

This, to me, seems to be a fundamental sticking point in the life balance and personal wellbeing thesis. As social agents we have scripted lives, which define how we *should* be in everyday life and prescribe, to a certain extent, the activities in which we *should* hold meaning or experience satisfaction. The difficulty arises when these 'shoulds' do not match with personal 'wants', because this creates incongruence between what we *actually do* and what we *want to do*, or who we *actually are* and who we *aspire to be*. The gap between what people *want* to do and what they actually *have* to do in everyday life can lead to psychological stress or ill-health because the incongruence they perceive between the two leads to a lack of satisfaction, self-worth and a coherent sense of self or personal identity. As Kofodimos puts it, our sense of self is formed through:

> An image of a person that we want to be and feel we should be... The image always incorporates a set of 'shoulds'; who we should be; how we should be; how we should feel; and what we should want. Furthermore we seek to live up to this image, and our self-esteem depends on how closely we feel we are living up to it. The problem with this dynamic is that the idealized image does not match the range of dimensions of our real selves. (1993, pp.59–60)

WHAT ABOUT IF YOU LIKE WHAT YOU ARE DOING?

It might appear from what I have said so far that obligatory activities are all bad, but in fact this is not so; it seems that the things people *want to do* can include the obligatory activities in life. Indeed some people love their work and get immense satisfaction from it; Huw was a perfect example:

> I mean certainly myself, I guess I've always strived to progress and make things better. Hard when you work for departments where, maybe people aren't quite so, you know, not as driven or motivated. I do find that difficult. But that's my personality. Whether I'd be playing, I don't play cricket for England or whatever, but that would be me. If I took a hat trick I'd, yes, I want it fourth down [laugh].

Other people, like Arial, love being a mother and she seemed to achieve that meaningful occupation without experiencing major conflict between the roles of paid work and home:

> I'm a mother first and foremost... I love being a mother... It might sound a bit weird but that's who I am. Like I said earlier, I do my best at work but that comes second. It always has and it always will.

Now both these stories support Hakim's (2006; 2007) notion of preference theory and both individuals seem to have made 'genuine choices' (Hakim 2006, p.287) about how they wanted to structure their work–life balance: Huw is obviously work-focused and has actively chosen that path; Arial is clearly home-centered, but has also chosen to participate in paid work in a part-time capacity. So what was their life balance like?

Huw was a married man, with no dependents. He viewed paid work as his meaningful occupation and had few or no interests beyond his chosen career; consequently, he experienced few, if any, conflicts with his home or social life because his attention was unilaterally focused on work. Arial, on the other hand, was a married woman with children and valued this role as her meaningful occupation. To maintain this attention on her family she made a deliberate choice *not* to progress in the workplace and believed that, through making this compromise, she had found her balance in life:

> I'm a [junior grade] and have been for God knows how many years. And I've been part-time because I've not really applied for anything else. Because it suited me to stay that grade. And I think I made the choice. Was I going to go all out being sort of aggressive or an ambitious career woman or whether I was going to have my priorities as my family? And I think people do. They find out their balance. And maybe people do go for their career and the family

might take second place. I think with me work has definitely taken second place.

Although both Huw and Arial described themselves as living a reasonably balanced lifestyle, there were notable consequences in relation to their choices.

Huw's choice

Huw was work-focused to the exclusion of everything else and his meaningful occupation was dominated by a drive for achievement. His identity and self-worth was shaped by participation in paid work and there was no sense of self, personal meaning or passion beyond that one occupation. Consequently, however meaningful his paid work might be to him, this was not a balanced lifestyle: it was a unilateral, exclusive focus on one activity.

Now whilst Huw described no sense of loss in this lack of variety in his life, he did identify frustration, real genuine angst, that others in the workplace were not as determined and driven as him to succeed. He also described feeling immensely dissatisfied by his position because he felt he should have achieved a more senior position by this point in his career, even though he was, in fact, progressing well. Perhaps the most telling point in Huw's tale was that he recognized himself that he could never fulfill his own desires, because his performance orientation was so strong, achieving one goal would never be enough – he would just strive for another:

I'm not completely fulfilled. Maybe I have to be a little bit more patient in time but even if I was head of the service, it wouldn't be enough. I want to be head of the [whole organization]. But I think that's me.

Now if Huw has made his choices freely, should we judge them? Maybe not; yet by his own admission there was little or no satisfaction in his life, just a continual drive to succeed. With no achievement ever being enough, then when would his life be paced and when would life be restive, restorative and spiritually enriching? When would he achieve a sense of fulfillment and personal meaning? There is far more to life than just paid work and putting all one's time and energy into one basket can create instability. Jamie, another of the occupational therapists who took part in the study, described this beautifully by using the analogy of a ship at sea:

Think of your life as if it's a ship. If you've got lots of different compartments and there are various different cargos, such as different activities and roles you have in your life, then if you have a leak in one it's not so very significant because you have all the other bits to keep you afloat. The moment you start losing that balance, that diversity of things that are interesting and valuable to you, that's when life tends to get more out of balance and then you start to sink and go under.

To achieve wellbeing through balance then, there has to be more to life than just a unilateral focus on one activity, such as paid work, even if this *is* your preferred occupation; you need a variety of roles and occupations to help you keep afloat and adapt as you progress through life and deal with life challenges (see Figure 3.1). If you do not do this, then you risk sinking and going under; as Arial put it, 'I know lots of people who've worked long hours and are really fabulous at what they do, but they've not done anything outside [of work] and when they've retired they've died; because they don't know what to do with their lives.'

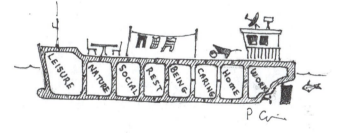

Figure 3.1 The ship of life

Arial's choice

Arial is a Welsh name that means courage. It was a pseudonym I gave to this lady because she was so very resolute in how she lived her life and I came to admire her immensely; I learnt a great deal about living a life in balance from Arial.

As I described previously, Arial had made a clear choice to put being a mother first in her priorities; yet she did engage in paid work and had done so for many years, carrying both roles (and all three associated shifts) throughout her working life.

She had always worked part-time and had genuinely made that choice to participate in paid work, yet she felt guilty: guilty that she did not do the long hours that others did; guilty that she could not stay on and extend her working day when requested to do so by others (because commitments at home prevented it); guilty that she had not progressed through the traditional promotion hierarchy and fulfilled social expectations.

She told stories of others remarking she was 'weird' because she had not progressed to senior positions, of 'emotional blackmail' to stay longer at work to complete requests to see clients and finally, she identified a latent worry about the decisions and choices she, herself, had made:

> Maybe if I'd made the opposite decision there would have been... probably there would have been conflict. And I probably would be divorced, I think, if I'd made the opposite decision. Or I might have, you know, made the decision I wasn't happy with it [prioritizing being a mother] and probably feel awful or upset then that I hadn't risen in the ranks. But then I think a lot of internal talking and then you can justify things to yourself, and be happy with that I think.

For Arial, the choices she had made were situated in family values and did fit with these (although you may read hesitation in her words above), but these choices did not sit well with a career. She was happy with this; they were her values too, but the element of doubt, the *what if* was there: what if I had built my career... would my life be different?

Then there were the attitudes and values of the others in the workplace, which differed from her family network and consequently classified her as 'weird'. Arial found this challenging and described disliking feeling 'different'. She was distressed that she felt pressed for more commitment in terms of working hours and evidencing ambition in the workplace; she resented this and found it demoralizing. This led her to question her own decisions, worrying whether or not she had done the right thing by making the choices she had, even though she was living her life in the way she wanted to, because others made her feel it was wrong.

When you consider these experiences, then you see that the option to make choices in the neoliberal workplace is possible, but, and this is the critical issue, they are shaped by social boundaries, expectations and opportunities; reflected in the eyes of significant others in the workplace and the values and expectations of our family networks. Consequently, they are never truly free, and can only be genuine if they match or fit with the external, socially driven ideal and the internal, personally modulated meaning.

Huw's choices, in first light, may seem to do this, but he was not living a really meaningful life: he had compromised that in order to live his career, and that is not a balanced lifestyle choice. The workplace did not object to Huw's decisions because he was so work-centered, but how influential these choices were to significant others or activities outside of work or to his own wellbeing over time were concerning.

Alternatively, Arial's choice to prioritize being a mother was disliked by others in work because this did not fit with social expectations or organizational ideals; consequently she worried about their views and compromised promotion to keep her workload manageable. This shows that although both these life choices were bounded by social expectations and have unintended consequences, Huw's choice was the most valued in social and organizational terms, and this is the critical issue about choice: essentially, there should be a place for both of these career paths in the workplace and one should not be prioritized over the other in terms of value, promotion or respect. Both should allow for a life beyond work because a career, however meaningful that might be, should not exclude living a balanced life. This leads us onto another interesting dilemma – what happens about life balance if you are not in paid work at all?

TO WORK OR NOT TO WORK, THAT IS THE QUESTION

In neoliberal capitalism paid work is the ultimate priority and the most important role in life. So what happens if you do not take part in it? There could be several reasons for this. There may, for example, be barriers that prevent you accessing the workplace, or you may be unable to find a job; you may be retired or you may have decided you do not want to work. Whatever the reason, you have a problem; either you are not achieving the expected norm, or you lack the kudos that comes with it.

So what do we become when we do not work? The answer is variable depending on your reasons for not working, who you are as a person, and how your support networks and social circles respond to this; but in general we either fill up our lives with other obligations of the non-paid kind to fill the void, promote non-obligatory activities into the realms of obligation, or at the other end of the spectrum become detached, de-motivated and under-committed. I would like to look at two different scenarios to unpick how these kinds of responses can occur.

SCENARIO 1: OVER BUSY AND RESENTFUL

Ruby had worked full-time in a professional job all her life and had brought up a family. She was now divorced and retired. Her children lived nearby and she frequently cared for her grandchildren to support her son, daughter and their respective spouses to participate in paid work. She felt this was something she *ought* to do, first because she no longer worked and she was their mother/grandmother and second, because she could see the stress this caused her children and wanted to help. She reasoned that she did now have the time to do this, because she no longer participated in paid work and consequently she had 'free' time to help.

Ruby, however, also did do voluntary work driving for a local charity, transporting community dwelling older adults and disabled people in the area to appointments or to the shops; through her church she also did regular spells in the local food bank.

Now when you look at Ruby's activities you can only feel admiration. She was really putting back into her family and community networks, and there was a real sense of self-worth and personal satisfaction from what she did; but she was also exhausted and felt more than a little resentful about the amount of time and energy she found herself giving to others.

So what was going on here? After all, she was not in paid work and had not been forced into doing these unpaid activities, so why was she not living a more balanced life? Using Schaef's (2004, p.22) descriptions noted in Chapter 1, Ruby was a 'busyaholic'.

Simply, Ruby was giving too much to others and had completely forgotten to build in time to care for herself. She now felt obliged to continue to do these things and felt unable to cut down her commitments because it was *expected*. The fact that she felt compelled to continue caused her to feel very frustrated, because she loved painting and drawing and had been looking forward to developing these skills in her retirement. Unlike the experiences shared earlier in this chapter, Ruby was not over-obligated in paid work but she was over-obligated in unpaid work and for her, the conflicts that arose between maintaining that and achieving her personally meaningful activities felt as real as those who experienced conflicts between paid and unpaid obligations.

SCENARIO 2: UNDER-BUSY: DISENGAGED AND UNHAPPY

Jake was 21 years old and unemployed. He lived at home with his parents and claimed job seeker's allowance (benefits to support people to find paid work in the UK). This meant he was fit and able to access paid work, but sadly, he could not find a suitable position. He had been unemployed since leaving college at 19 and although he had worked part-time in a bar throughout his studies, he now needed a higher paid, more permanent position that could offer a living wage. This was proving difficult to find and was having quite challenging consequences.

He found that not earning money really impacted on the quality of his life because he could not afford to access even the simplest of activities he enjoyed. These included socializing in the pub, going to the gym and airsofting (shooting BB guns). Consequently, he spent most of his time playing computer games in his bedroom and was very demotivated, depressed, irritable and apathetic; he could see no positive future or purpose in life. Jake's problem was, in one sense, quite the opposite of Ruby's: he was under-active, not engaging in meaningful or productive, purposive activities at all and disengaged from life.

However, a common trait he did share with Ruby was that he too could not access activities that were meaningful to him, even though he was in the enviable position of having the time to do things he enjoyed. This was because, frustratingly, he did not have the money to do it. He was under-obligated in both paid and unpaid work and this meant he was time rich but money poor.

What these scenarios show is that it is not only paid work that can cause conflicts or imbalance in life with other obligatory and non-obligatory activities. You can over-commit to obligations outside of paid work or fill up your life with other activities and over-commit to them; consequently, you still do not have the time or means to access the things that are meaningful to you. Alternatively, you can detach from life's commitments as Jake did, and lose a sense of worth and self-esteem to such an extent that you withdraw from any type of purposive activity at all, but still not spend time in meaningful pursuits. These scenarios identify how important paid work or unpaid obligatory tasks are to identity, self-esteem and self-worth, but also illustrate the need to balance these meaningfully with a variety of doing, being, belonging and becoming activities.

CONCLUSION

To me, challenging Hakim's (2006, p.286) thesis of having 'genuine choices' in how paid work is balanced with life, there appeared to be very few genuine options for those who were working and had families to care for, or those who had to carry out domestic responsibilities. In all cases there were real consequences or compromises because the ideal patterns of paid work were, if not for full-time (which was definitely the preferred), certainly *full-on* commitment to the workplace with policy, practice, social thinking and organizational cultures all overlooking other life goals. This exclusive focus on paid work was not nirvana even for the driven, work-centered individual, because they too had to give their all to the workplace to the exclusion of building a meaningful life outside of work, and whilst that could seem OK for some, it was the death knell for a rounded life balance marked by participation in a variety of doing, being, belonging and becoming activities: neoliberalism is not just an economic system but also a cultural one, demanding full commitment, without distractions (zero drag), in whatever hours one participates in the workplace, and this culture creates life imbalance, irrespective of the outcomes on individuals and their family or community networks.

Interestingly, for those who do not participate in paid work there is no respite; for them, the drive to overcommit is transferred to unpaid obligations and non-obligatory activities are morphed into the realms of obligation. Self-importance, value and self-esteem, it seems, are still the measure of success and the shoulds or 'oughts' of life remain the ultimate priority; compromise, in terms of loss of personal meaning which in reality is the most important activity of all, is an accepted loss. We will return to the importance of the 'ought' self in Chapter 5 and meaningful activities in Chapter 7.

CHAPTER 4
STRESS, BURNOUT AND RUST-OUT IN LIFE IMBALANCE

INTRODUCTION

Stress is a growing problem in our modern lives and is affecting not only our physical and subjective or emotional states of wellbeing as most research suggests, but also our psychological, social, ethical and spiritual dimensions of health. It is perhaps unsurprising that much of this stress is clearly linked to lifestyle imbalance and, as our overwork and over-busyness continues unabated and unhindered, so this type of stress is becoming chronic, resulting in exhaustion or burnout and another less known, and in one sense counterintuitive condition, the so called 'rust-out', a term coined to encapsulate a state of apathy and disengagement from life activities, a little like Jake who I introduced you to in Chapter 3.

Key to these kinds of stressors are the social and cultural contexts, values and expectations we, as people, impose on each other and ourselves in our everyday lives and consequently the complexities of the networks and relationships we live and work in. These include our social, family and workplace networks, as well as the larger communities and political and socio-cultural networks in which we are embedded.

Significantly, there are also other elements at play in how we experience stress from over-busyness and disengagement in life, including how we respond to that stress and what coping mechanisms (if any) we utilize. This relates to our unique repertoire of skills and personal strategies, as well as our individual personalities and attributes.

Although our unique personalities are a part of who we are as individuals and, consequently, how we deal with our everyday lives, it can often be difficult to ascertain how that impacts on what we do, because our own level of self-awareness about how we react and respond to certain stimuli and view certain situations can be limited or deceptive. This is why some of the thought management and mindfulness techniques that will follow in Chapters 5 and 6 are so useful in finding a personally meaningful life balance: because they help us to identify what we are thinking about, review who we are and understand what we really want from life.

Now whilst our own thoughts can sometimes be difficult to grasp and understand, perhaps even lower in our everyday level of awareness is the natural physiological responses that occur in the body when we experience stressful situations or stimuli. We do, of course, all know about the well renowned human fight, flight or freeze (fright) response that kicks into action at times of stress, but do we understand how it biologically happens and why we can also experience a state of longer term or chronic stress?

For those of you with little knowledge of this response, I will give a brief overview to contextualize the ensuing discussions. Please note, however, that this book will not give you a comprehensive account of the physiological components of stress and consequently those of you who want a more detailed description might want to supplement your reading. Robert Sapolsky's (2004) *'Why Zebras Don't get Ulcers'* is a recommended read, although there are a variety of suitable texts available on the subject to suit all tastes.

THE PHYSIOLOGY OF THE HUMAN STRESS RESPONSE

The human stress response is part of a complex interconnected network called the nervous system, which is composed of the central nervous system (CNS), including the brain, the spinal column and the peripheral nervous system (PNS), which connects the CNS to the rest of the body and environmental stimuli.

At the most basic level, the PNS is divided into two main systems: the somatic or *voluntary* nervous system that controls our active 'doing' activity, and the *involuntary* or *autonomic* nervous system, that works more in the background, ensuring we do things like regulate our body temperature through dilation or constriction of the blood vessels and activation of the sweat glands. You may have heard the term *homeostasis* or *allostasis* to describe this important function in terms of regulating the body to adapt to changing stimuli.

In terms of the human stress response, it is the *autonomic nervous system* that does most of the work. This system has two branches, the *sympathetic* and the *parasympathetic,* which work in opposition. These two branches can send signals to all parts of the body to influence how we feel and act in times of stress, the former eliciting the fight, flight or freeze response so we can deal with threats, and the latter inducing a more relaxed state when safety is assured and the threat has passed.

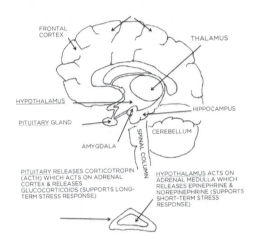

Figure 4.1 How the brain orchestrates the stress response

The part of the CNS that orchestrates the stress response is the *hypothalamus* in the brain (see Figure 4.1). When a stress trigger occurs, the hypothalamus sends signals to two parts of the body: the *adrenal medulla* in the adrenal gland and the *pituitary gland* in the brain. The adrenal medulla acts directly on the *autonomic nervous system* and activates the *sympathetic branch* to kick into action to produce the fight, flight or freeze response. This means we can run off at speed or fight with that inhuman strength you can sometimes muster when you really need to.

At the same time, the pituitary gland acts on the adrenal *cortex* and works not only to support the action of the sympathetic branch, but, by releasing different chemicals, *sustains* that action over much longer periods (see Figure 4.1). This continued action is key to maintaining periods of long-term or chronic stress and consequently has an important role in conditions such as burnout and rust-out, as well as more general stress experienced through life imbalance. I will now explore the stress response in more detail so you can understand how it works in relation to life balance.

THE AUTONOMIC NERVOUS SYSTEM

As mentioned, the autonomic nervous system (ANS) is part of the peripheral nervous system (PNS). It has two branch lines and is a complex, interactive network of hormones and neurotransmitters (chemicals) ensuring we do automatic things to maintain allostasis.

The ANS stimulates the stress response by acting upon the *endocrine system,* exciting this to secrete a variety of chemical messengers. As mentioned previously, the autonomic system is controlled by the brain and this is a very important point to bear in mind (no pun intended!) because although much of the stress response is automatic and is predominantly *unconscious,* there are some actions that can occur in *conscious* thought, which means that we *could* potentially have some sense of control over it and consequently manage it. We will examine these elements of control further as we progress through this chapter and the rest of the book.

THE TWO BRANCHES OF THE AUTONOMIC NERVOUS SYSTEM

You are already aware that the ANS has two branches called the *sympathetic* and *parasympathetic.* The parasympathetic branch has quite a different effect on the human body than the sympathetic, and the two work alternatively in a dynamic dance of opposition, which means that only one or the other of the branches is active or in control at any one time. Through this synergy they orchestrate the human stress response, and the exchange of control from one branch to the other is very important because it causes major changes to how we feel and behave.

At the most basic level, the sympathetic branch instigates the acute stress response, so at times of danger, or when we *think* there might be danger (here is an important bit about the brain being in control… we *think* there might be an danger), we can fight, run or freeze in the hope of saving our lives.

When the threat has passed, the sympathetic system slows down and eventually stops, knocking off the acute stress response and allowing it to dissipate. This process assures the sympathetic branch has time to build up its chemical reserves and prepare for future action, but also enables the parasympathetic branch to switch on, stimulating a more restive and relaxed state, something we need to do to maintain our physical, emotional and psychological balance. In order to understand this process, I will now describe what makes the branch lines knock on and off and intermittently change over (see Figure 4.2).

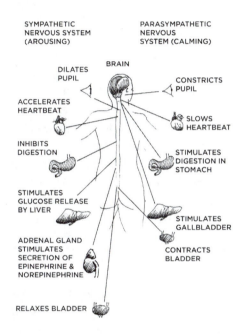

Figure 4.2 The sympathetic and parasympathetic branch lines

The sympathetic branch

During these times of actual or *perceived* danger, the sympathetic branch of the ANS activates the production of *adrenaline* or *epinephrine* in the adrenal glands (found above the kidneys) and this releases adrenaline into the body (see Figure 4.2).

Adrenaline has several different effects on the individual, but at the simplest level, it puts the person on red alert and predisposes the body to be ready for that fight, flight or freeze response. It does this by influencing several part of the body such as accelerating the breathing, speeding up the heart, constricting the veins, dilating the arteries, increasing blood flow, pumping more oxygen around the body and pouring glucose into the muscles to prepare the body for action (see Figure 4.2).

In addition to adrenaline (or epinephrine), a veritable cavalcade of other hormones are also produced and get into the stress response scrum, including *noradrenaline* (or *norepinephrine*), *glucocorticoids* from the adrenal gland, which act as the back-up to the adrenaline, *glucagon* from the pancreas, and *endorphins* from the pituitary gland and brain, which pump sugars (energy) and pain relief respectively into the blood stream.

For primal humans this kind of response was of course a very necessary tool. In times of acute action, when, for example, you needed energy and strength to fight or hunt and kill food, or alternatively in times of danger or threat, for example, when you needed to run because perhaps you were on the menu, it would have kicked into action and possibly served to save your life. But today, whilst the physiological response remains much the same, the stressors we experience tend to be very different. At lunchtime, for example, it is not necessary to hunt and kill a mammoth to satiate hunger, but queueing in the coffee shop and worrying about whether you will be served in time to get to your next appointment can stimulate the same physiological stress response; whilst we do not have to run miles and attack our enemies to get to our hunting grounds, driving the car on our modern congested roads is a very common precursor of road rage, which is, of course, the old fight response getting into play.

Similarly, feeling overwhelmed by too much work (paid or otherwise) and dealing with difficult people or situations can activate the stress response, which, depending on your personality and the situational factors at the time, can augment some rather inappropriate responses in the social context: you get mad in a meeting and say something you regret and storm out; you freeze up when asked a question, say nothing and look like a rabbit caught in the headlights; or you try to avoid certain situations by ducking into doorways every time that certain person walks by.

Now the problem with these kinds of responses in modern life is that they are not effective: situations are not improved by verbally attacking someone in a meeting, freezing up, ducking into doorways and closets, or running away from work pressures. First, this is not socially acceptable, and second, it just does not solve the problem but rather maintains the stress cycle (see Figure 4.3).

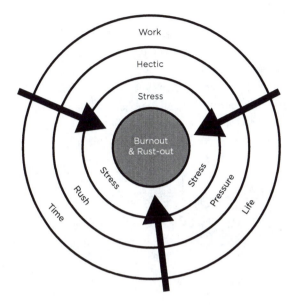

Figure 4.3 Stress cycles in everyday life

So what do we do with our raging stress response in our 'civilized' world? Well, and this is the crux of the bludgeoning levels of stress we have in our so-called modern societies, we sit on it; and that leaves us in a bit of a conundrum. Before I explain this further, let's look at the action of the parasympathetic branch of the ANS because this is key to re-establishing a sense of calm in our busy lives.

The parasympathetic branch

Now you will remember that as the sympathetic branch gets you into action the parasympathetic does the opposite. It does this in a couple of ways. In common with the sympathetic branch, the *parasympathetic* is set in motion by the brain and it stimulates the release of various hormones and neurotransmitters that act on the organs of the endocrine system. However, in this response, it releases a very different cocktail of chemicals with very different kinds of results. In particular, it produces *acetylcholine,* inducing a sense of calm, promoting a relaxed and restive state and stimulating physical growth, energy storage and a general sense of wellbeing and optimism, conducive, I would suggest, to the state experienced during participation in 'being' types of activities. This system slows you down and facilitates a sense of balance and harmony in life. This is why the two branches cannot be active at the same time: because they actually oppose one another in the chemicals they produce and subsequently in how they make you act and feel. This means if you can elicit the parasympathetic system to switch on, you can knock the sympathetic branch off and you can experience a more relaxed state (see Figure 4.4). Think of it like driving the car; you cannot accelerate and brake at the same time because the two actions cancel each other out, so if you brake slowly and calmly you will eventually slow down, feel more in control, and be able to stop, breathe and relax.

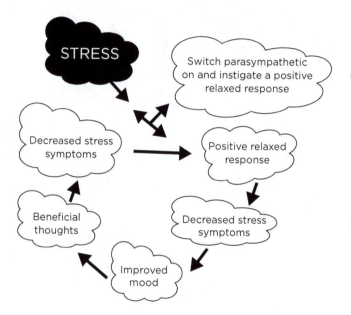

Figure 4.4 Putting the parasympathetic into action:
The positive relaxation cycle

SO WHAT HAPPENS IF THE SYMPATHETIC BRANCH NEVER SWITCHES OFF?

In terms of the stress response, if the sympathetic nervous system does not switch off, your stress levels will increase and can eventually become chronic. Over time, this can have quite profound results, leading to disease, exhaustion, burnout and/or rust-out and eventually extreme ill health.

This happens because at a physiological level we have activated the sympathetic nervous system and it has stimulated that lovely cocktail of neurotransmitters and stress hormones which are coursing through our veins at 100 miles per hour; we are raring to go but there is no-one to fight and nowhere to run to or hide, so consequently we do not burn off that cocktail of chemicals causing that pent up energy as our ancestors would have done.

When those chemicals remain in our body it leaves us feeling physically or emotionally tense over much longer periods of time. The sympathetic system builds up into a crescendo of hyperactivity and the parasympathetic branch remains switched off, preventing the relaxed state we so crave kicking in; and that leads to first acute, then chronic stress (see Figure 4.5).

Coming back to the car analogy, if the engine is never switched off and travels at 100 miles per hour, it will eventually become frazzled and exhausted, and will ultimately burn out, break down then rust out.

If you are in this chronic state of stress, what can you do to overcome it? Well, you need to get the parasympathetic branch in action and this means, you've guessed it, more restive, *being* types of activities and time to do things that are meaningful and enjoyable to you; otherwise you will remain permanently stressed, and this leads to lots of problems, not only physically but emotionally and psychologically. The emotional and psychological context is of particular concern in terms of life balance because when we cannot fight or run to burn off angst, we do tend to store lots of negative thoughts in our heads and consequently feel more and more worried (see Figure 4.5); and worry is a dark master in life imbalance.

THE TROUBLE WITH THINKING: WORRYING AND MEMORY

The capacity of the human being to feel and think about stressful situations leads to a second unfortunate problem that occurs in our rather more socially constrained and structured modern age, and that is the capacity to worry about everyday things that *might* occur: traffic jams *might* make you late for work, an important meeting or to pick up the children from school; what *might* happen in meetings because of a difficult relationship at work and what *might* happen if you do not achieve your performance outcomes.

This ability to imagine the worst scenario (catastrophize) and anticipate or imagine stressful events that might occur (the crystal ball approach) means you can experience and maintain ongoing *psychological* and *emotional* as well as *physical* stress.

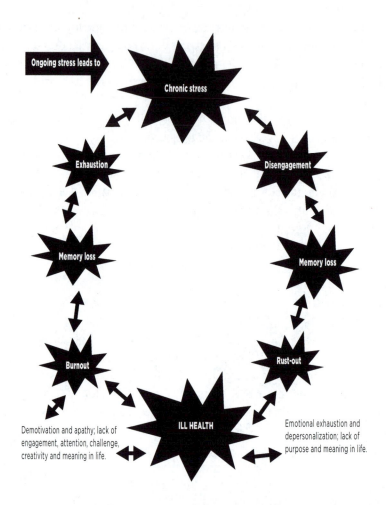

Figure 4.5 The chronic stress cycle

As you will recall from the previous chapters, worrying about work (paid or otherwise) was an extremely common type of stress response for people, with ruminating thoughts and disturbed sleeping patterns underpinning physical and emotional ill-health (see Chapter 2).

Notably, this kind of 'stress in the head' has as much to do with how we *think* and *feel* about stressful situations and what we *imagine* might happen as it does to the physiological responses. This is the thinking bit of the stress response that I mentioned at the beginning of this chapter; because the brain is worrying about these *potential* events, so the natural physiological responses are activated, working in anticipation of *possible* future stress scenarios (which may or may not become a reality), evincing a *chronic cycle of stress*, which we are perpetuating by our own thought patterns (see Figure 4.5).

WORRYING IN THE STRESS RESPONSE

When you are overworked, over-busy or just plain exhausted you can worry or ruminate about things. This can be at any time of the day or night, but can often be more apparent when you wake in the wee small hours or when you are trying to get off to sleep. Thoughts that during the day were niggling become huge, insurmountable mountains, everything is awful and you feel like you are carrying the weight of the world on your shoulders.

Now sleep is a very important restive and relaxing activity: it helps you feel well and replenish your stores of energy; it can promote wellbeing. The parasympathetic system is active when we sleep and helps to restore that necessary balance; but when you are awake and worrying, the sympathetic branch kicks in and keeps you awake, leading to more stress, more worry, more stress cycle (see Figure 4.5).

When you are *thinking* about a stressful event or worrying about something, those thoughts can cause the *hypothalamus* (see Figure 4.1), to activate not only the sympathetic nervous system, but also that second stress response I mentioned that stimulates the pituitary gland. This gland secretes a hormone called *corticotropin* or *ACTH* (see Figure 4.1) into the blood stream, and this in turn activates the production and secretion of hormones from the adrenal glands, called the *glucocorticoids*. These not only back up the sympathetic *adrenaline* and *noradrenaline (epinephrine* and *norepinephrine)*, but also have that longer lasting, more sustainable action I noted earlier. Consequently, in common with the implications of constrained physical release of energy and tension extending the physical effects of stress in the human body, so *thinking* provoking worrying can initiate and maintain the stress response over longer periods, again leading to chronic stress conditions but also profoundly impacting on our memory (see Figure 4.5).

THE MEMORY IN THE STRESS RESPONSE

There are times in life when the stress response can enhance memory, and there are other times when it does not. The simple reason for this is that when you have short bursts of mild to moderate stress this can, depending on the circumstances, enhance recall and sharpness effectively: think about doing exams or giving a paper at a conference. On the other hand, and this is the problem, long-term stress, precisely because it is *not* transient, has the opposite effect and tends to reduce it.

The trouble with protracted stress is that, whether you like it or not, having the sympathetic branch system permanently switched on, and the adrenal glands pumping out glucocorticoids, degrades the ability of the brain to store and retrieve memories as effectively as if the sympathetic and parasympathetic were more harmonized (balanced) in terms of which was in control at any one time.

So in terms of memory, what is going on when the stress response is permanently switched on?

The complexity of memories

I am going to keep this simple just so you have an idea of how it all works rather than giving you a detailed account, so do bear in mind when you are reading this that our brain is far more complicated than this simple summary suggests.

You will probably be aware that the brain has a *long-term* and *short-term* memory storage facility; what you may not know is that we also store different *types* of memory. Here I am going to focus on three parts of the brain that have three different types of memory storage. At the most basic level, these are:

1. *Explicit* memory is concerned with storing facts and events and your conscious knowledge of that: who you are, what your family look like, what you enjoy and the day of the week. These tend to be sorted and stored in the *frontal cortex* and *hippocampus* (see Figure 4.1).

2. *Implicit or procedural* memory focuses on your skills, habits and knowing how to do things: when learning to drive a car you use the explicit memory initially, but once you have learned and practiced a little, it becomes more procedural or implicit; you carry this out without conscious thought, yet can respond quickly when you need to. These kinds of memory tend to be stored in the *cerebellum* (see Figure 4.1).

3. *Feeling and emotional memory* tends to be stored in a part of the brain called the *amygdala* (see Figure 4.1). This part of the brain works at a more *unconscious* level than the frontal cortex and the

hippocampus and it is this potent mix of unconsciously held feelings and emotions, including stress and anxiety, that makes the amygdala very important in the stress response.

What happens in these parts of the brain during stress?

You will remember than when we are under stress the body produces more glucose to fire up the body to get us ready to run or fight. Well that glucose also gets pumped into the brain and releases glucocorticoids to help us to form and retrieve memories; remembering how you got out of a sticky situation previously or problem solving quickly could, after all, save your life.

The trouble is that when we keep the stress response switched on over a protracted period, we produce too many glucocorticoids and the brain begins to get flooded with them. When this happens, the ability of the hippocampus and frontal cortex to retrieve and store memories starts to *decrease* and we lose the ability to either store or remember facts or actions, influencing explicit memory and the implicit in terms of the learning of new tasks. This is a common scenario we can probably all relate to: forgetting the name of someone you know you know when they are right in front of you; forgetting where on earth you put the cars keys; being asked something in a meeting and you cannot remember the answer even though you know you know it, and struggling to learn a new task.

Now the problem with this in terms of life imbalance is that at the very same time the cortex and co are feeling overwhelmed and losing the ability to recall and store memories, the *amygdala* is having a whale of a time, because it gets really excited by loads of glucocorticoids whizzing around, and it starts to remember and store *feelings* even more effectively. The trouble with this is that when the amygdala is in this hyper-effective state it stimulates you to remember and recall *feelings and emotions* to do with stress and anxiety, making the present situation much, much worse. If you have that niggling sense of fear and anxiety but cannot quite relate it the situation you are in, think about your amygdala; it may well be recalling past events and previous stressful situations and it is those feelings re-emerging that are making this situation seem so, so bad. This does not help with our thinking and feelings of stress in the present moment; indeed it has quite the opposite effect, building on our fears, concerns and worries, leading to exhaustion, burnout and rust-out (see Figure 4.5).

BURNOUT AND RUST-OUT

Studies have illustrated that life imbalance can lead to chronic stress and from there to states of burnout and rust-out. However, these are two very different conditions and it is worth explaining how they differ, because although both can arise from stress in relation to life imbalance, they can be quite markedly different.

BURNOUT

Burnout has been closely linked to *overwork* (paid or unpaid) in life imbalance and tends to be defined as a syndrome consisting of three dimensions: *emotional exhaustion*, resulting in the depletion of the psychological energy necessary for satisfaction in everyday life; *depersonalization*, resulting in negative attitudes towards significant others; a sense of *low personal accomplishments* and a belief that life *lacks purpose and meaning* (Edwards and Burnard 2003; Lloyd and King 2001) (see Figure 4.5).

As we have seen from previous chapters, this kind of feeling was very common among the occupational therapists that shared their stories about overwork. They described stress, exhaustion and a perception of life as just a little pointless:

> I find myself not having a full lunch break and working till 5.30–6 o' clock to try to get the work done. I've been just feeling exhausted. So 7.45 [am] till about 6 o' clock to 6.30 [pm] I'm out of the house. So I have four waking hours a day for my own time. So I get back at 6 o' clock. I go to bed at 10. Read till 10.30. 'Cos I'm too tired after. And go to sleep by 10.30.

Of course what is happening here is that the sympathetic system has been consistently switched on and is in hyper-drive; physiologically it is getting exhausted, as of course is the poor person, who at this stage is totally drained of energy. The problem is then exacerbated because when burnout (exhaustion) sets in, we rarely respond by knocking the sympathetic branch off and knocking the parasympathetic on (see Figure 4.2). Oh no! We push the sympathetic branch on, trying to do more and making the whole problem even worse, and then start worrying even more about what we have NOT done; 'I think I leave so many things undone and I go home obviously thinking about the cases and how is it that protection of this vulnerable adult hasn't happened.'

Because we are worrying, we get stuck in a negative pattern of thought and, consequently, cannot sleep. Where feelings of time scarcity are met with avoidance of restive activities such as sleep, leisure and relaxation, so that pushes us even more over the edge, increasing our sense of physical and psychological imbalance and feelings of being out of control; 'But I think that's coming to it. The problem. If you can't get balance, if you can't get sleep, you go crazy.' So what can we do? At this point we *have to* switch our parasympathetic branch on and rest even though that is the last thing we can envisage ourselves doing. If we do not, then we will begin to crumble and develop even more serious conditions such as depression and anxiety.

RUST-OUT

Rust-out is a condition that is specifically associated with lack of *engagement* or *attention* to particular occupations. It is often linked with a profound state of *demotivation* and sense of *routinization* in the paid work context, but is also relevant to other daily activities where it is associated with repetition of tasks, a lack of focus and/or stimulation, the lack of a challenge and, perhaps most of all, the loss of *creativity and meaningful engagement* to stimulate personal interest and enthusiasm.

As a key component of a satisfying life balance is linked to experiencing a *meaningful occupation* and *engaging* with, and being fully attentive to, at least some aspects of life (remember Csikszentmihalyi's psychic energy noted previously), then it is unsurprising that when this is lacking, people experience frustration and/or a lack of motivation, apathy or even boredom in life.

At its worse extreme, rust-out can result in complete disengagement from activities (remember Jake in Chapter 3), and sadly this kind of state can have very poor press, because it is closely associated with socio-cultural-political ideologies of worthlessness. For example, people experiencing this condition are frequently derided as those who (a) might not like work, or do not want to work or do their bit for society or (b) those who appear not to be engaged or motivated by work or any other social expectations. However, if we review those assumptions in the context of rust-out, it can offer a very different perspective on what is happening for some people in our respective societies, and how that state of affairs might have come about; it is a perspective worth thinking about and, consequently, I would like to explore disengagement in terms of life balance a little more.

The causal factors of disengagement

Imagine you are so pressured in work and so exhausted that you can no longer engage with (give focused attention to) your tasks in a meaningful way. This is a point where you might be beginning to experience rust-out, probably unconsciously, as a response to chronic or extreme acute stress.

Rust-out can also occur when you are *prevented* from doing something *you want to* do or when you are *forced* to do something you *do not* want to do, usually by some external force or barrier. In these situations your choice or self-determination over your ability to engage in something is either thwarted, coerced or forced and consequently is outside of your control (Carriere, Cheyne and Smilek 2008; Cheyne, Carriere and Smilek 2006).

Box 4.1 A tale of two rust-outs

a. 'And it's the routine of work wears you out. Every now and again I start to feel as if I'm on a hamster wheel. You know, I'm getting out of the bed. I'm getting in the shower at the same time. I'm slapping on the same makeup. I'm wearing the same suit. I'm getting in the car at the same time. I'm going down the same drive and going down the same motorway and seeing the same cars. And I'm going into the same car parking space. I'm not one for routine and it's enforced on you. So I find that quite stressful you know? I don't like that, you know… And what you start to do then, you start to cram everything into the weekends. And you know, I notice things I enjoy, like impulsive things don't happen any more.'

b. 'You can do things like take it [work] home with you. Or come in a bit earlier and work. But you don't want to start doing that really. Because it starts eating into your life. You've got to explain it to your partner. Or you don't take up the hobbies or go out and see your friends and stuff like that. So it [work] starts getting in the way there. And it does. Work takes up so much. It exhausts you. It makes you boring. If you're bringing stuff home at night, you're gonna do that first while you still got the energy. Everything then gets shifted to the weekend and that's a guaranteed failure really. I mean it really. So it's got a messy big F written all over it. Failed. Try harder [laugh]. I think, yes, I think that really impacts for me. Yes.'

Box 4.1 offers some examples of this: the occupational therapists identify that the pressures of paid work were *enforced* on them and they feel they have no sense of control; they also describe a lack of challenge and feeling *disengaged* from work, describing tasks as repetitive and life as *routine*. In these examples, tasks at work dominate life but the enthusiasm for them has dissipated; work has become boring because there is little or no challenge in it; rather, it is mundane. Life has become fixed and routinized because there is no time or energy left after work to do activities that are *personally meaningful*, even the simple ones like spending time with friends. In essence, there is no time or energy or the will (*intention*) to do being, belonging or becoming activities, and that takes away the dynamic interconnectedness of a balanced life.

When you consider that a satisfying life balance in everyday life is found in (a) having personal choice and control over your participation in activities; (b) accessing personally valued or meaningful activities; and (c) feeling challenged by and engaged in activities, then it is unsurprising that disengagement can influence life satisfaction and, consequently, balance and wellbeing in quite profound ways.

Csikszentmihalyi (1997) has intimated that when life is so busy we disengage from certain activities, a process of re-engagement can be stimulated by introducing tasks that are more challenging because we have to think about them and give them focused attention, which means we *engage* with the task, even if it is something that is not personally meaningful. This is a top tip in overcoming disengagement and I will return to this later in the book.

CONCLUSION

To summarize then, stress and chronic stress conditions like burnout and rust-out can all be symptoms of life imbalance. These symptoms can arise because you have too much to do and/or are overworked, but other factors are also at play. First, where there is no sense of control or *personal autonomy* over managing workloads (paid or unpaid) and where you feel pressured to do something you *do not want* to do, or prevented from doing something *you do want* to do, you will also feel stressed because you are not accessing activities that are personally meaningful or achieving personal goals. Second, when you do not give your full attention to activities because you are stressed or because you have no time and energy to do so, so you lack the ability to *engage* in it and that decreases your satisfaction and effectiveness in that activity and, subsequently, increases your levels of stress. Third, in modern life the underlying physiological stress response to environmental stimuli, the fight, flight and freeze response, is activated in times of life imbalance; where the sympathetic branch of the autonomic nervous system stays switched on over long periods, chronic stress conditions will develop; *glucocorticoids* will remain active in the body, stimulating the amygdala to keep remembering previous stressful situations in both thinking and feeling contexts, resulting in heightened states of stress and anxiety.

All these interconnected factors underpin how you feel and experience life imbalance and can profoundly influence your sense of wellbeing in everyday life.

So what can you do? In terms of the physiological responses, you need to learn to keep the parasympathetic branch switched on and running gently around the track. This means you have to recognize when you are stressed and knock the sympathetic branch off; you need to use time and energy for participation in meaningful activities and balance doing things with being, belonging and becoming pursuits, because they facilitate the parasympathetic response. You also need to inject *creative tension* into the workplace, that is, a dynamic dance between challenging tasks and the more normative everyday workplace activities, which are achievable but hopefully not too mundane, to facilitate opportunities to *engage* in tasks, even if they are not personally meaningful. The following chapters will offer you some ideas about how you can do this.

PART 2

MOVING FROM 'DOING' TOO MUCH TO RECONCILING BEING, BECOMING AND BELONGING

CHAPTER 5

FINDING LIFE BALANCE
Strategies for Change

INTRODUCTION

This chapter is the first of the second part of the book which aims to offer the reader practical ideas to living a more balanced lifestyle. The following chapters do not claim to have the perfect solutions, because life balance is a very complex and interconnected phenomenon, but they do offer techniques to think differently about how you approach and view your life balance and share strategies to facilitate living in a more personally fulfilling or harmonious way.

To begin this journey I will start by exploring the importance of your personal sense of self: your knowledge and understanding of your own self-identity and why that is essential to finding fulfillment and satisfaction in your own life balance. If you think about it, this is common sense: if you know who you are and want you really want from life then you will feel more fulfilled, and consequently, experience a greater sense of meaning and wellbeing in life.

It is perhaps unsurprising that this apparently simple suggestion is not as easy as it seems. In our busy lives we frequently forget about seeking personal knowledge and meaning in life; these kinds of existential questions are parked on the side whilst we run around doing whatever it is we think we *need* or feel we *have* to do.

These drives toward doing are intricately interwoven with the sense of self and, in part, shape our identity, highlighting how social, political and cultural concepts are integral to our understanding of who we are because they profoundly influence it.

In this chapter we will explore how these different influences interweave to form the multiple facets or dimensions of the self; as individuals we truly do have many faces.

Now this journey of discovery is, of course, just one step toward change and living your life differently. Consequently, the ensuing chapters will support this quest by exploring how we can be more mindful in everyday life (Chapter 6); how we can think about time differently to achieve a sense of personal meaning in life (Chapter 7); how we can establish a sense of personal autonomy over life balance even in cultures that intensify imbalance and in situations in which others have more power than us (Chapter 8), and finally, how we can think about life balance in a more interconnected way (Chapter 9). In this sense we end up with a mix of different strategies that we can use in synergy to grow and sustain a more balanced lifestyle in everyday life.

A SENSE OF SELF: KNOWING WHO I AM AND WHAT IS MEANINGFUL TO ME

Knowing who you are and what you really want out of life is really important in understanding what your ideal everyday life balance looks like; but answering those questions is not necessarily easy because we do not spend much time really thinking about them. To begin to explore this, we will consider first what a sense of self or self-identity is, and then how we can begin to get to know our true 'self' a little better.

THE SELF-IDENTITY

Our notion of our self-identity or 'self-concept', namely, the knowledge, feelings and assumptions we have about ourselves is complex. It is shaped by many factors including by our relationship with the social and natural (or external) worlds, our perceptions of how we see our inner self or selves (our personal inner world), and how those worlds interact and the congruence or incongruence between our view of the 'self' and how others see us. This means the sense of self is both multidimensional and interconnected: a product of many parts. Yet it is also mutable because we have a temporal nature, we grow older; the human consciousness means we can learn, feel, think, adapt and become more than our present selves. In fact it is this very ability that is the basis of personal growth, i.e. the capacity to fulfill one's potential and self-actualize or be all that you can be in life.

This may sound a little complicated, but I will now explore these different aspects of the identity in more detail and describe how they are relevant to our life balance. Critical in this context of life balance are the relationships and congruence between the *ought, ideal* and *actual* selves, the *past, present* and *future* selves and the *relational* selves.

THE INFLUENCE OF THE OUGHT, IDEAL AND ACTUAL SELVES ON LIFE BALANCE

The actual, ideal and ought selves are aspects of the self-concept that have a profound influence on life balance. The *actual* self is the representation of the attributes you, as an individual (the personal/internal facet), and/or significant others (the external/social facet) *believe* you do *actually* hold: this is you acting and being in the everyday context (see Figure 5.1).

Alternatively, the *ideal* self is composed of the attributes that you (internal/personal) and/or significant others (external/social) would *like* or *hope* you will become and correspondingly, also represents the person you and/or they would *least* like you to become, i.e. the feared self (see Figure 5.1).

Finally, the *ought* self is the representation of the attributes, specifically in terms of responsibilities and obligations, that you believe (internal/personal) and/or significant others believe (external/social) you *should* hold. It carries the sense of duty and obligations you feel that you *have to* do every day and is strongly shaped by what others expect of you; this is the self that says; 'I think I should be doing this' (see Figure 5.1).

Now the problem with these three aspects of the self is that they do always coalesce and to add to this conflict can be incongruent (discrepant) in a variety of ways. First, as I have described, each of the aspects of the self has two faces: the one *you think* you have or want (internal/personal) and the one *others think* you have or *should* want or have (external/social), and these two faces can either match (be congruent) or differ (be incongruent or discrepant). For example, *your viewpoint* about your ideal self, or what you want out of life and what *others expect you* to become or want can be different. Alternatively, the things *you think* you ought to do and the things *others think* you ought to do can also be congruent or incongruent (discrepant).

Second, the three aspects of the self need to be in harmony with each other if you are to feel in balance or congruent in life. For example, your ideal self (the aspirational or becoming self) and what you actually do every day (the actual or real self) may be incongruent because your hopes and aspirations do not match what you are actually doing in your everyday life. For example, you have to work and be busy to such an extent that you cannot fit in the piano or gardening, which is your ideal activity; or your actual and ought selves may be incongruent because you cannot fit in all the work or caring commitments you want to because there is just not the space to do it (see Figure 5.1).

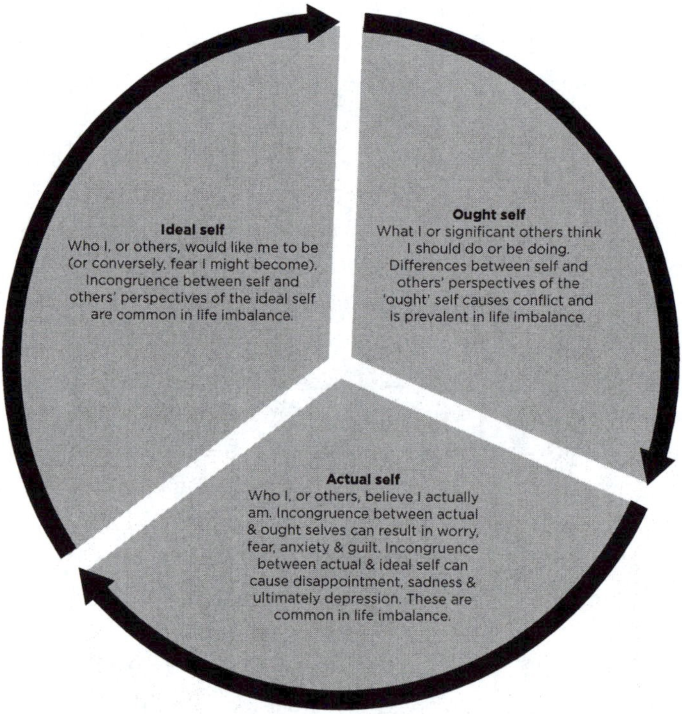

Ideal self
Who I, or others, would like me to be (or conversely, fear I might become). Incongruence between self and others' perspectives of the ideal self are common in life imbalance.

Ought self
What I or significant others think I should do or be doing. Differences between self and others' perspectives of the 'ought' self causes conflict and is prevalent in life imbalance.

Actual self
Who I, or others, believe I actually am. Incongruence between actual & ought selves can result in worry, fear, anxiety & guilt. Incongruence between actual & ideal self can cause disappointment, sadness & ultimately depression. These are common in life imbalance.

Figure 5.1 The ought, ideal and actual selves

As I have discussed these possible discrepancies, it has probably become clear that these multiple selves are influenced by stereotypes and the socio-cultural-political structures that surround our everyday lives and shape our expectations, values and behaviors. The problem with this is that in neoliberal economies both the ideal and actual selves are strongly shaped by the ought selves. Think about it: I or you *ought* to be in paid work; I or you *ought* to be busy; I or you *ought* to be managing all my/your commitments/ obligations; I or you *ought* to be personally responsible. Consequently, these 'oughts' can become the things to strive for, sublimating the ideal self and identifying what the actual self *should* be doing.

But what if *your* image of your ideal self is something else, or you sit outside of that perfect 'ought' image for some reason? This is a huge problem because *your* image of your ideal self is what *you want to* strive for to fulfill your potential and that is thwarted. It is perhaps unsurprising then, that if you experience this kind of incongruence or discrepancy, whether it is between two or more of your three aspects, or between your personal expectations and the expectations of others (the external/social), then you can often feel less fulfilled, more conflicted and consequently imbalanced in life.

Now that might seem complicated enough, but there are also other dimensions of the self that shape our self-identity and are part of who we are. We all have a biography or life story: a past, present and future self, if you like; and we are all *relational* beings, 'entangled with significant others' (Andersen and Chen 2002, p.619) because we exist in and of networks and complex relationships. These multiple facets of the self have implications for our 'self-definition, self-evaluation, self-regulation, and most broadly for personality functioning, expressed in relation to others' (Andersen and Chen 2002, p.169). This means we have many other dimensions of the self which shape our unique personality to consider before we can understand a little more about who we are and how this self-concept influences our life balance.

PRESENT, PAST AND FUTURE SELVES

The ought, actual and ideal selves are in part a product of, and further complicated by, our notions and understandings of our former selves: our past and upbringing (who I was/where I came from); our present selves (who I am now, my current traits, beliefs and values) and our possible future selves, identified by our goals, aspirations, hopes, fears and fantasies about the possible future (who I can or could become). Working together as a whole, the past, present and possible future selves intertwine to provide a sense of biographical continuity: a consistent 'me' over time if you like, and create a schema or framework through which we see our 'self' and understand our everyday experiences. This is about your personality; your unique self.

The ideas we hold about our future selves are important for two reasons. First, they reflect our belief in our potential and consequently motivate and incentivize our present behavior (what I need to aim for and what I need to avoid) and second, we evaluate our present selves in light of these imagined futures and find ourselves achieving or wanting.

Since future selves are not manifest but rather *imagined*, so they are most vulnerable to the possibility of change and can potentiate different futures in response to present occurrences; if our self-concept is shaken by present events then the future self can become more negative and vice versa. How you respond to these events can also be influenced by your personality and traits: 'An optimist is a person who extrapolates possible selves on the basis of positive current experiences, whereas a pessimist extrapolates possible selves on the basis of negative current experiences' (Markus and Nurius 1986, p.966). This is your cup half-full and cup half-empty scenario.

Now of course, whilst as individuals we are free to develop a multitude of possible selves and make personal choices about who we are and who we want to become, these identities are, like the ought, ideal and actual selves, shaped by the socio-cultural-political context in which we are embedded and the values of significant others in our life domains. Our upbringing can have powerful influences over how we see the world, how we function and respond to our natural and social environments, and how we envisage our potential, and can also characterize how positive or negative we are about our future. In essence, these aspects of the self can shape our personalities and identify the values we hold about paid and unpaid work, our families, our self-esteem, self-worth and drives. Thus, how others have influenced us over time is relevant to who we become and how we respond to and react in our everyday dance of life balance, as well as how we measure our success in our socio-cultural life and our worth in our work or family performance. This leads on to the importance of the relational self as a dimension of self-identity.

THE RELATIONAL SELF

If you think about your life in terms of the relationships and interactions you have with significant others (people with whom you have close, emotional relationships or who are significant in your life) you will recognize how those relationships have shaped your individual personality, both in your childhood, as you constructed a core sense of identity, and then throughout your life, as you grow, because the actual, anticipated or remembered evaluations and concerns of significant others are continually organized into your working self-concept (Markus and Nurius 1986). This means that the sense of self is shaped by the expectations of, and interactions with, others, and acculturates self-worth as a measure of achieving specific social norms or outcomes in small, significant groups or settings, as well as in wider socio-cultural customs (Andersen and Chen 2002).

Relational selves are closely associated with a sense of belonging and therefore are an influential source regarding how we reflexively identify the necessary interpersonal patterns of behavior to be accepted (or indeed rejected) by those near to us, and consequently are intertwined with the past, present and future selves as well as supporting the ideal and ought selves, which are connected with those wider relationships embedded in social structures.

The relational self is a powerful contender in the personality stakes; it is a potent force in creating our emotional and motivational relevancies, in building our individual differences, and consequently underpins how we, as people, can respond differently to life situations including how we cope with and dance out our own life balance. From these descriptions it is probably becoming very clear how incongruence in these multiple aspects of the self-identity (see Figure 5.2) can influence your life balance, and I will now offer some possible scenarios.

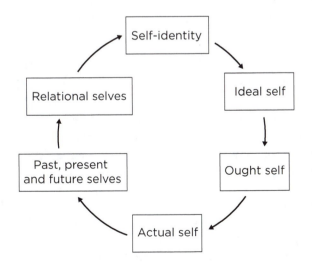

Figure 5.2 The cycle of multiple selves influencing self-identity

WHAT DOES THIS MEAN FOR LIFE BALANCE?

As I have already mentioned, when the ideal self (who I or others *want* me to be), the real or actual self (who I am or who others *think* I am) and 'ought' self (who I or *others* think I *should* be) are compatible or *congruent* with each other, then you will live a more balanced lifestyle, because you will feel you are being and becoming who you want to be. However, when you broaden your understanding of the self-concept to encompass the other aspects or dimensions of the self, you recognize that you also have to achieve a sense of harmony with these other facets, including the past, present, future and relational selves, if you are to attain a positive sense of wellbeing in terms of life balance, and this is about how your personality and relationships can underpin a state of imbalance. Let's look at this in more detail.

INCONGRUENCE BETWEEN THE OUGHT, IDEAL AND ACTUAL SELVES

In terms of life balance, it is very easy to confuse the ideal self with the 'ought' self and lose out on the actual self as a consequence. This happens because social drivers and norms suggest to us that paid work, for example, is the most prestigious activity to participate in and consequently we put this first, irrespective of our own personal values and meaningful activities. Worryingly, we often do this because we think this is the right thing to do. These means we compromise, often unwittingly, those things we value or want to do the most by striving for socially valued goals, and may even convince or dupe ourselves into believing these occupations *are* personally meaningful to us. Handy described how he fell into this kind of trap and explains how he experienced a loss of purpose and self-esteem as a consequence:

> The problem was that in trying to be someone else I neglected to concentrate on the person I could be. That idea was too frightening to contemplate at the time. I was happier going along with the conventions of the time, measuring success in terms of money and position, climbing ladders which others placed in my way, collecting things and contacts rather than giving expression to my own beliefs and personality. (1997, p.86)

Accounts like this challenge us to see beyond the symbolic and social capital of paid work and indeed the notion of obligation located in the unpaid obligatory tasks we do every day, to see ourselves differently and accommodate into our lives our own personal interests. This is not an easy task because we are constrained and shaped by expected norms and we also have strategies for self-protection, including self-delusion, which prevents the need to confront ourselves in terms of living a more balanced lifestyle, but as Handy points out, you do have a real self that deserves to be let out. So what can you do in this situation?

Find the real you: The actual self

As mentioned earlier, the actual self is the real you and is, in part, shaped by your values, passions, talents or skills. Finding this self and being honest about who you are in life will provide a space to be more creative and fulfilled, if you can accommodate the time and energy to spend in activities that you find personally meaningful and resonate with your intrinsic values. By being true to yourself and knowing who you are, you have a grounded sense of self that you can be centered by and return to when life throws you off balance (Wheatley 1999). One of the occupational therapists I spoke to described this as follows:

> If you want to have a balance you can work it out I think. Usually you can negotiate with people and work it out. But if you want to be a workaholic and work all the hours you can make that choice as well. And pretty much if you stress yourself out like that then it's down to you to make that decision and to let people do that to you or do that to yourself ultimately. You need to be yourself as well rather than just the various labels that you have as you go through life. And have a chance, you know, just to be what you want to be.

Now the challenge, of course, is the actual self is not only complicated by the ideal and ought selves, but by the past, present, future and relational selves, who can convincingly divert you from your preferred path and so challenge this process of self-regulation.

THE PAST, PRESENT, FUTURE AND RELATIONAL SELVES

I have already described why knowing who you are is very important because this provides that grounded point in which you can find your center when you are thrown off balance; but how your personality has been shaped by others is vital to understanding how you, as an individual, respond to life imbalance and what strategies you use to establish balance in your life.

Sian, one of the occupational therapists I spoke to, talked about how her relationships with her parents (significant others) and her childhood experiences with them (relational self and past self) had influenced her behavior and attitudes to work:

> I think I am a perfectionist. I think I have just naturally, through my upbringing and background, got very high expectations of myself and I think other people have got them of me.

This learned behavior, this adopted attitude, made her work harder and longer and created stress and imbalance in her life.

Mhari, another of the occupational therapists, described how her present relationships in her family meant she was expected by her significant others to carry the full domestic load, even though she now worked in paid employment. She was unhappy with this situation and wanted to change it, but felt unable to because, prior to taking on paid part-time work, this was the way things had always been done (past self), and this pattern met the obligations and expectations of the family (relational self and ought self by others). As these were now taken-for-granted aspects of her everyday life (actual self) and were embedded into the aspects of her the daily interactions with significant others (relational selves) they were hard to challenge and change and Mhari accepted this; 'I know that a lot of it is my fault because I have always done it, you know. And his mother always did it. He [husband] never did anything at home before we got married. I always... I did it you know. So.'

Clearly then, the sense of life balance we have is intricately linked to who we are, and in common with that sense of self is reflected a complex web of perceptions held by self and others, shaped by interactions over time, which may or not be congruent with who we think we are or want to be. One could suggest that life balance is an essential aspect of the sense of self because how we interact with life is through activities and how we make sense of that life experience is through dimensions of meaning; consequently, the search for balance is, in part, a search for self and meaning in life as these three things, balance, self and meaning, walk hand in hand.

THE IMPORTANCE OF PERSONALITIES IN SEEKING LIFE BALANCE

If balance, self and meaning are integrated, then knowing who you are and what is meaningful to you is key to finding your personal sense of balance, and consequently fulfillment and wellbeing, in life. So to begin this section,

I want you to think about your personality type in terms of how you deal with life balance.

IDENTIFY YOUR OWN PERSONALITY TYPE

Now you will have probably heard of several different ways of categorizing personalities and you may well have had a go at some of the questionnaires or tests available to do this. I am not going to ask you to do anything as complicated as that. I just want you to think about how you respond to your life balance; how you think about what you do in your life and whether any of the following descriptions resonate with you.

The 'aholics'

You may recall from Chapter 1 that Schaef (2004, p.22) has identified that in our over-busy world people can develop obsessive or addictive tendencies about being busy, becoming workaholics, rushaholics, busyaholics or careaholics, all of whom 'do' obligatory activities in life to the exclusion of anything else. Now I have certainly been a workaholic and recognize that aspects of my personality and upbringing brought me to that point. However, I have met others who fall firmly into one or more of the other obsessive behaviors and these patterns dominate their lives, eroding meaning, engagement, balance and wellbeing. So what about you? Can you see yourself in any of these behavioral patterns and if so, what aspects of your personality brought you here? (see Figure 5.3).

Now an important point to consider here is that although the 'aholics' tend to be very driven, addictive or obsessive-compulsive types (Huw in Chapter 3 is an example of a workaholic), in our over-busy lives the need to develop one or more of these behaviors in order to cope with the high level of obligations and busyness is far more prevalent than in societies or cultures that *do not* drive overwork and busyness as the norm.

The Careaholic
You get overly involved with others and worry about them constantly, forgetting about yourself. You over-empathize to such an extent that others' emotions become your own; when you are not caring for others you feel bereft and have no other interests beyond that task; you get satisfaction from committing to and caring for others; you may suffer from burnout or exhaustion as result of over commitment but you continue to place this as your priority activity. In essence, you have filled your life with belonging activities and have forgotten the rest.

The Workaholic
You think about work all the time and engage in work all the time, and it subsumes all other aspects of your life. Whatever you do, work is there and you are thinking about it. Consequently, you are not engaging meaningfully with others, or any other being, becoming or belonging activities. Your 'doing' activities are focused around work and you may be experiencing exhaustion, burnout or rust-out.

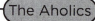
The Aholics

The Busyaholic
You are constantly on the go; if you are not working (paid or unpaid) then you are doing something else, even if that is watching TV, playing computer games or shopping; you have to do something...anything to keep your mind occupied. You like to be busy and hate being bored, yet you cannot engage meaningfully in any of your constant doings. This is a technique to distract your mind from thinking about the important things in life, like relationships, community, meaning, spirituality, joy and quiet; in fact any being, belonging or becoming activities are sidelined. It prevents balance and wellbeing. You may be experiencing burnout or rust-out.

The Rushaholic
You tell yourself to speed up; worry about what you have to do next; rush off and forget things; eat on the move; fail to notice what is going on around you and rarely notice beautiful things or nature; you finish other people's sentences and cannot sit still, often tapping your feet or fingers. In this behavior, your mind is so occupied by thinking about the next task, it is not in the moment and you cannot engage or be fully present in any activity, good or bad; consequently, this behavior thwarts engaging meaningfully in being, becoming or belonging activities and prevents balance and wellbeing. You may be experiencing burnout or rust-out.

Figure 5.3 Workaholic, rushaholic, busyaholic and careaholic
Adapted from Schaef (2004), p.22.

This is a notable point, because it means that Western economies push levels of addiction; but it also means that those of us who do not walk the obsessive path or do not love work, busyness or speed exclusively can still get forced into adopting certain strategies in order to survive.

Now this can be an unwitting adaption, or you may notice it happening and either fight against it or try to avoid it completely. These individual differences in how we respond to these pressures are due to our unique personality traits, which are, of course, a reflection of the multiple selves we dance with every day. So if you do not fall into the obsessive or addictive personality type and do not want to utilize that coping strategy, or if you do not love working constantly, or being busy, or you hate rushing around like a headless chicken but find that it is enforced on you, what do you do? Hochschild (2008, pp.85–88) has identified five different time management or *temporal* strategies that she believes people use to deal with busyness and overwork in terms of life imbalance. These strategies do, to some extent, support those offered by Schaef (2004), but rather than obfuscating with personal obsession, suggest strategies that are adopted when external pressures create over work and over-busyness and we have to cope somehow; in these circumstances, she believes we adopt behaviors that can be classified as the Busy Bee, the Endurer, the Deferrer, the Outsourcer and the Resister (Hochschild 2008, pp.85–8).

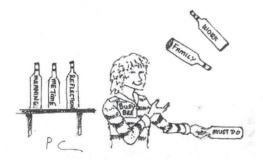

Figure 5.4 The Busy Bee

Busy Bees

I have started with the Busy Bee because this resonates so closely with Schaef's (2004) vision of the busyaholic and rushaholic. If you are a Busy Bee then you see the busyness of life as a challenge to be overcome and do this by actually embodying or incorporating a speeded up lifestyle into your self-identity and everyday routines; you are constantly busy, actually feel energized by the ensuing pressure, and love it. Your identity is wrapped in the fast pace of life and you gain satisfaction from that. You are not prepared to let anything go and do it all; you just divide life up into the necessary time packets to make it work and juggle with joy.

Now of course the problem with this kind of temporal (time) strategy is that you are so busy being busy, you have little or no time to just be, or become anything other than busy. You may do family tasks and caring and even do it well, but what about the feeling and emotional context? What about the time just to be a family, a parent, partner, lover or friend? When do you stop spinning, look, listen, hear and respond with feeling? When do you see beauty, feel the wind or smell the sea? This kind of life ends in burnout or rust-out because you exhaust yourself, or lose any sense of meaning or purpose in life, and just exist rather than live.

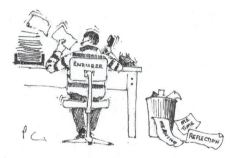

Figure 5.5 The Endurer

Endurers

If you are an Endurer then, according to Hochschild (2008), you manage the pressures and conflicts in your life balance by compromising personally meaningful pursuits to get the obligatory tasks done. If you are using this temporal strategy, you might feel you exist in a daily round of everyday routines and habits. You may love your family and care about them, but you may also feel you cannot engage with them in the way you want to, that is, meaningfully, because you do not have the energy, attention or time to do so. You might feel exhausted and overburdened, and if you stay in this state for any length of time you might start to experience exhaustion.

Many of the occupational therapists I spoke to used this temporal strategy to cope with everyday life and it was marked by conflict, compromise and predominantly burnout, but for some rust-out as the routinized nature of life became so repetitive and staid they began to detach from it. This is not a good way to live your life and requires an injection of meaning, passion, joy, excitement and spontaneity to make it worthwhile.

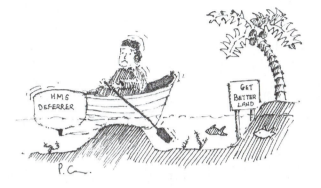

Figure 5.6 The Deferrer

Deferrers

If you are a Deferrer then you will believe the situation you are in will get better. It might be bad now, and yes it is stressful, but this is just for now; later, and this can be months or years later, it will improve. This is a different perspective from the Endurer, who accepts things are as they are, because the Deferrer sees light at the end of the tunnel and feels the conflict situation is temporary not permanent. River, an occupational therapist, for example, described how she saw her loss of meaningful activities and promotion at work as a transitory phase en route to her child growing older and therefore not needing so much of her time and energy resources: 'I know it will come back; you know in time that it will come back and I will be able to commit more to my own personal goals that I'm missing at the moment.' The trouble with this kind of strategy is that 'Get Better Land' is never actually achieved.

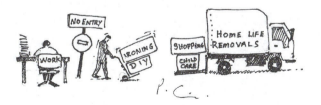

Figure 5.7 The Outsourcer

Outsourcers

If you are an Outsourcer you will do just what it says on the box: you will go to other people to support you with the activities you cannot fit in, including the meaningful and interesting ones. This can be caring for the family, as well as domestic chores, and when it includes the former, according to Hochschild (2008), it has to include excellence in the quality of care in order make the Outsourcer feel as if they can continue to give love to those they care about. This kind of idea resonates with the notion of quality not quantity in terms of the time you can give to your children, and is related to the sense of guilt we all carry when we are forced into this coping strategy. This was a technique used by many of the occupational therapists in the case studies, especially those who were part of a dual career couple working full-time. In reality, of course, like many of the other coping strategies, the choices available to working parents are all a double-edged sword with, yes, methods to support in managing work and life commitments, but none of which feel truly adequate.

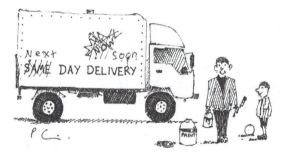

Figure 5.8 The Resister

Resisters

If you are a Resister, then instead of adapting to the demands and schedules thrust upon you, you alter them, or at least try to take it down a gear and not get wrapped up in the drive to be busy, to meet demands, buy others time or defer happiness until some future date. No, you will adapt your life situation to achieve what you want to do and attain the best outcome for you, even if this means you do not always flourish at work because you are not tied up with the need to chase the dream of success.

As Arial has shown us (see Chapter 3), if you are a Resister then, unsurprisingly, you will tend to be happier and have a better quality of life than Endurers, Deferrers, Busy Bees or Outsourcers, but you might have to compromise, and compromise a lot, to get what you want in terms of balance in life. Nonetheless, resisting is a sound strategy to adopt in seeking life balance in the present work-mad and over-busy world.

Now that you know what your temporal strategy is in terms of how you are managing life balance, the next stage is to think about whether or not you need to adapt or change it to achieve a more balanced approach to life. The problem with this is that in order to modify how you behave, you have to review how you *think* and *feel* and this is not an easy task, because in general we have little or no awareness of our thoughts and even less recognition of how they underpin what we do and how we respond to external events (review discussions in Chapter 4 if you need to refresh your memory about this). So what can you do to get to know your thoughts a little better?

GETTING TO KNOW YOUR THOUGHTS ABOUT LIFE BALANCE

Thoughts are a fascinating and very powerful means of influencing how you feel about your life balance and how stressed you are in life. The basic assumption is that your thoughts and beliefs can act upon and influence your feelings and actions (Beck 1976). Of course there are different types of people and different ways of viewing the world: some have a glass half-full approach, others a glass half-empty. Depending on this perspective, one can view the same situation very differently, and consequently it is your unique interpretation of an event that underpins how you feel and react in any one situation and, in this sense, there is an element of choice in how you respond to stimuli and how you can manage it (Neenan and Dryden 2011). There are different techniques to 'manage' or raise awareness of your thoughts and to either challenge or change how those thoughts might be affecting your everyday sense of self, performance and life balance.

Changing your thoughts

You may recall from Chapter 4 that thoughts can emerge spontaneously or in response to particular stimuli. They frequently work in the background, are often subliminal, or are noted merely as white noise or mental chatter. Where these thought patterns are negative and recurrent, you can become trapped in a spiral of negativity, which can stream unchecked through your mind (see Figure 4.5). The more negative these thoughts become, the more stressed they will make you feel and that frames how you enact your everyday doing, being, belonging and becoming activities and, fundamentally, shapes your experience of life balance. The problem with this is that if these thoughts are left to have free reign and are unchecked then they will, in essence, impact on how you behave and feel in your everyday life; so the question is how do we manage them?

Theories such as cognitive behavioral therapy (CBT), relaxation therapy, thought stopping techniques, meditation and mindfulness can all offer strategies to help you gain control over these negative thoughts in order to improve the way you feel. I will talk about mindfulness in the next chapter, as I do believe this has a specific affinity to life balance, but here I want to discuss the cognitive therapies, namely, those that actively capture your thoughts and change how you think as an effective tool in managing life imbalance.

COGNITIVE THERAPIES

Cognitive or thinking therapies (CT) have many forms, including cognitive behavioral therapy (CBT), cognitive behavioral coaching (CBC), thought stopping techniques and relaxation therapy. They all work on a similar underlying principle, and that is that negative thoughts can occur automatically and that these can be addressed and changed. These thought patterns are sustained by distorted beliefs or errors in judgments, which can be categorized in a variety of ways. Table 5.1 gives examples of negative and distorted cognitive patterns that are common in our everyday thinking about life balance. Read these through and see if you can identify any of these negative patterns of thinking in yourself.

Table 5.1 Negative or distorted cognitive patterns in life balance

Cognitive distortions	Definition
Overgeneralization	Based on one or a small number of events an individual draws unwarranted conclusions, which have wider negative implications. *'Management see us as a small and whining group and they **all** just ignore us.'*
Catastrophic thinking	Where an over-generalization is amplified to extreme proportions. *'This is a nightmare. If I don't start getting enough sleep I will go **crazy! I'll end up losing my job, my home, everything!**'*
Maximize and minimize	The tendency to exaggerate negative experiences in terms of daily activities, events or interpersonal relationships and minimize the positives. This is about making actual happenings seem worse than they actually were/ are. *'He was really horrible to me in the meeting. He **hates** me. It's because I supported the merger. He's **never** liked me and **he's out to get me.**'*
Absolute or black and white thinking e.g. all or nothing thinking	Unnecessary placing of complex issues into two possible polarized extremes in terms of outcome. Situations are viewed in either/or terms. There is no in-between: *'Either I **can** achieve a successful work–life balance or I **can't** and I'm a **complete failure** at it'.*
Mind reading	Drawing conclusions on the basis of inadequate information e.g.: *'My boss didn't email me back. **She thinks I'm a waste of space.** I know she doesn't like me.'*

Cognitive distortions	Definition
Crystal ball gazing or fortune telling	Pessimistic view of things that **might** occur: 'Oh my God. The boss has called me to the office. I just **know** this isn't going to turn out well!'
Personalization or taking the blame (remember personal responsibility-taking in Chapter 2? This is a symptom of it – seeing the self as **the** responsible agent)	Instead of labeling only the behavior, you attach the label to yourself, e.g. 'I failed to complete the job, so that makes me a failure'.
Selective negative focus or mental filter; ignoring the actual evidence	Undesirable or negative events, memories, or implications are focused on at the expense of recalling or identifying other, more neutral or positive information. Positive information may be ignored or disqualified as irrelevant, atypical, or trivial. This is the glass half-empty approach: 'There's no point talking about managing my life balance because **nothing will change; it never does**. So it's not worth trying really because **it won't make a difference**.'

Adapted from Beck *et al.* (1979) and Friedman, Thase and Wright (2008).

If you recognize yourself in any of these examples, then try the following:

- Step 1: recognize them as distortions or errors in judgment and accept that they bend the truth or reality of the situation.
- Step 2: begin to revise how you think about that situation.
- Step 3: identify a more accurate and evidence-based appraisal of events which is more accurate and positive and could facilitate a move towards self-management and resolutions.
- Step 4: put that accurate and more positive pattern into action.
- Step 5: review and repeat the process.

Now whilst research has shown that cognitive therapies can be as effective as medication in treating stress, depression and anxiety, all of which occur in life imbalance, in order to benefit from these techniques you need to commit yourself to the process, and that is not an easy pledge to make. A therapist or coach can help and advise you, but they cannot make your problems go away without your full co-operation; this means you have to *want* to do it. Once you make that commitment, then hopefully you will benefit. Some simple techniques to support these steps for you try yourself at home follow.

THOUGHT STOPPING TECHNIQUES

Thought stopping techniques are a key technique to change how you think about your life balance. If you consider the five steps I noted earlier, you may have wondered how you could stop the negative thoughts from reoccurring and yes, although repeating the five steps would help, there is another method that is very useful in doing this, and that is thought stopping techniques. So what are these and how do you do them?

You will recall that I spoke about the mental chatter or white noise in your head which, if you pay attention to it, can turn out to be very negative thoughts that underpin how you think and feel, and that if you capture those thoughts, review them and adapt them into a more realistic or positive pattern, so your wellbeing will improve. Well, thought stopping techniques support this by helping you to break that negative cycle.

Take, for example, some of the common negative thought patterns voiced in Chapters 2 and 3: waking at night continually mulling things over about work, or visions of being hamsters stuck on incessantly turning wheels and wanting to shout 'stop' and jump off. Both these scenarios provide perfect examples for when you can find thought stopping techniques useful.

In the first, for example, when you wake at night, you might visually imagine yourself pressing a red stop button or jamming the cogs of worry, ending those persistent and negative thoughts, and then replace that undesirable pattern with a more positive or realistic evaluation of the situation. In the second, you might actually envision yourself slowing your speed down gently on the wheel (like on the treadmill in the gym), jamming it with a plank of wood or, if you are a real dare devil, jumping off... that one would not work for me... I'd panic! So the image has to suit you and mean something to you; it is an image about being in control or having some sense of autonomy over your own thinking and feelings about life balance and, if you remember, autonomy is a key tool in finding your own life balance.

Sometimes your thought stopping techniques can need re-enforcements to help break the negative cycle or maintain the new pattern of thinking. Remember that once negative patterns have been established they can be darn hard to change because your mind automatically switches on to them whenever you are stressed (remember the amygdala in Chapter 4) and as long as the sympathetic nervous system remains on, you are stuck on that negative track. This is where relaxation and deep breathing techniques can help.

RELAXATION AND DEEP BREATHING TECHNIQUES

Sometimes the thought stopping techniques need a little help to break the cycle by switching the sympathetic track off and the parasympathetic track on. Learning relaxation techniques can support this because, as I described in Chapter 4, if you are relaxed you cannot be stressed and in a relaxed state you can think more positively and feel more in balance.

A key stage in understanding how to relax is to learn how to breathe. This is not as daft as it sounds because most of the time we do not breathe deeply. When you are rushing around, enduring, deferring and even resisting you are active and using energy. Often, as part of this, and particularly when you are stressed and the sympathetic system is switched on, you breathe shallowly to conserve your energy (go back and take a look at Figure 4.2). When you breathe shallowly you breathe into the upper quadrant of the ribcage, which increases or maintains the stress and tension you hold in the body. To counteract this you need to learn how to breathe deeply into the abdomen, because this can switch the parasympathetic branch of the autonomic nervous system on.

To practice how this feels try lying on the floor or bed and inhale through your nose; feel the breath traveling down into your lungs and notice how the ribcage expands, first at the level of the breastbone, then at the level of the diaphragm and finally, how the breath flows into the abdomen and how that rises to accommodate that life-giving breath. When you breathe out, breathe out through the mouth; first the abdomen will fall, followed by the lower then upper part of the ribcage and finally, that stale air from your body will be expelled.

Box 5.1 runs through this process using a simple three breath approach; the more often you practice this technique, the more you will benefit and learn how to relax. Over time, this technique can enable you to facilitate feeling relaxed in even the most stressful situations.

> **Box 5.1 *Three breaths to deep breathing***
> - Close your eyes if you can.
> - Focus on the breath and inhale through the nose and exhale through the mouth.
> - Lengthen your breath for a count of three:
>   - breathe in through the nose for the count of three
>   - hold the breath for the count of three
>   - breathe out through the mouth for the count of three.
> - Pause for one normal breath.
> - Repeat until you have completed the cycle three times.
> - Resume normal breathing.
> - If it helps you, say this mantra in your mind:
>   - when I exhale I breathe out stress
>   - when I inhale I breathe in serenity.

There are many forms of relaxation, and what you like and which method you use is basically a personal choice based on preference or possibly need. Jacobson or progressive muscle relaxation, for example, is a good method to use if you are not aware of how it feels to be stressed or how it feels physically to hold tension in your body, because it guides you through this: first tightening (to become aware of tension) and then letting go (to become aware of relaxing) different muscle groups in the body. This is followed by guided visual imagery to help you relax your mind. The best way to do this is to envisage you are either in a safe place you know or somewhere imaginary: in a beautiful forest, at the beach listening to the waves, or sitting on a mountain top and feeling so free your thoughts just melt away.

Autogenic methods, on the other hand, rely more on your own mind letting go of your tension and embracing relaxation. For example, you might begin by imaging your toes, and then your whole right foot, are feeling very warm and comfortable; you imagine the foot is feeling heavy and very, very relaxed; you then move up to the lower leg, and imagine that too is feeling warm and relaxed; then move to the upper leg and then repeat the process in the left foot and so on. Following completion of this process for the whole body, you again let the mind relax by imagining yourself in a safe and beautiful place of your choosing and just letting yourself dance in the peace and tranquility of it.

There are literally hundreds of examples of these types of relaxation techniques on YouTube, and many are also available as apps for your phone. If you use one of these, this means you can run through the whole process with your eyes closed, lying or sitting in a safe, warm and comfortable room where you will not be disturbed. Alternatively, if you want to use the practical advice offered here to create your own relaxation practice, you will need to remember the steps and use the power of your own mind. Whatever you decide, ensure you practice somewhere where external disruption is kept to a minimum: shut the door, unplug the phone, place your mobile on silent or flight mode and play gentle and soothing music if that helps. The world will still be there when you return, but the colors will be richer and life will seem just that little bit calmer and kinder.

CONCLUSION

To summarize, you can make a difference to your own life balance by getting to know yourself and understanding your own personality and coping strategies in life. You can develop techniques to adapt these, to breathe, relax and keep the parasympathetic branch of the autonomic system switched on. You can engender a sense of autonomy over your own thoughts and make your thinking positive, learning not to ruminate on the past, which can lead to depression or to worry about the future, which can result in anxiety. By utilizing these strategies your life can feel more fulfilled and balanced. However, another key element to remember in life balance is that one of the most important relationships of your 'self' in your life is the relationship with the now, the present moment, and this is the focus of the following chapter.

CHAPTER 6
MANAGING LIFE IMBALANCE
Living in the Moment

INTRODUCTION

In this chapter I will talk about mindfulness, or living in the moment, which at its most basic level is a technique to move from constant *doing*, or busy states of mind and body, to *being* more present in the moment by having a physical, emotional, psychological (cognitive) and spiritual awareness of self, in time and space, as it unfolds.

In terms of reviewing thoughts and feelings, mindfulness differs quite dramatically from the cognitive therapies discussed in Chapter 5, because no attempts are made to evaluate thoughts as rational or distorted, to change thoughts judged to be irrational, or to reduce unpleasant emotions associated with thoughts; rather, cognitions and emotions are simply noted and observed as they come and go. In mindfulness, thoughts are as seen as thoughts, as mental events and no more, a creation of your over-busy (and consequently *mindless*) mind; and whilst you should become aware of these thoughts (be *mindful* of them) and even name them if that helps, you should then let them pass you by, like clouds scudding in a rolling sky or ripples sailing in a flowing stream (Kabat-Zinn 1990). Consequently, mindfulness is an important technique in achieving life balance because it supports people to move from the normal state of busyness: doing too much, worrying about the future, or ruminating on past events; in essence, having a mind so preoccupied or full of thoughts, it is totally unaware or *mindless* to the moment, to drawing our attention to, and being fully aware or *mindful* of, and embedded in, the present moment (mindfulness), so people experience life differently (see Figure 6.1).

This chapter will offer practical techniques in mindfulness to help you to understand how you can achieve this different sense of time and experience it in terms of life balance, and to consider how you can become aware of, and then let go of, your everyday life stresses. You will hopefully learn how to use these techniques in everyday situations and to apply them in all life domains, both inside and outside of paid work.

It is worth noting here and now, that mindfulness is not necessarily an easy state to achieve, but neither is it impossible. People do have the ability to learn and apply these techniques to their everyday lives; but what is extremely hard to do is to break the regular or habitual patterns and routines that dominate our everyday doing and change them in order to integrate the techniques of mindfulness into our daily dance of time and energy and then regularly practice them so they become the norm.

A key tool for success in terms of using mindfulness to support your own life balance is to adopt three key elements in terms of your own thinking and approach to practice; these are *intention, attention* and *attitude* and I will explain what these mean and describe how you can do this in detail later (see Figure 6.2).

To begin our journey we will start by understanding mindfulness and its influence on life imbalance, then explore some basic techniques we can use to overcome these situations in everyday life to facilitate achieving a more harmonious state of balance and wellbeing.

WHAT IS MINDFULNESS?

Mindfulness is something you have probably heard of: it is now a very common word in the public domain and is associated with living in the present moment, as it actually happens, as well as being in harmony (balance) with yourself, others and the natural environment.

This is quite different from our usual, everyday state of affairs. Consider, for example, how often do you get out of the car and realize you have no recollection of passing a certain spot or even driving down a certain road? How often do you have no memory of where you have put your car keys, your glasses, your wallet or purse? How often do you worry about whether or not you have locked the front door, turned the iron off before leaving the house, or even where you have parked your car in the car park? The reason we forget these things is because we are preoccupied with our thoughts: worrying about being late, where we are going, what we have to do next, either later in the day or even next week, or ruminating about the argument we had with our partner that morning.

These daily worries populate our minds and mean we are either constantly agonizing about something that has already passed or fretting about something that might occur in future. By occupying our minds with either past or future worries or concerns, so we become oblivious to the *present moment*. Where this is underpinned by too much work or too much busyness, so we can fall into the 'aholics' syndrome I discussed previously (see Figure 5.3) and become obsessed with 'doing'. Alternatively, you might adopt the coping strategies described in Chapter 5 to deal with the pressure: enduring the pace under duress, becoming a 'Busy Bee'; speeding your whole self up, dragging significant others with you to embody the pace; continually telling yourself it *is* going to get better sometime (Deferring), even if, in reality, that is highly unlikely; paying others to do your home life (Outsourcing) or finally, Resisting the pressures and somehow doing it your way, even though that can sit uncomfortably with others (see Figures 5.4–5.8).

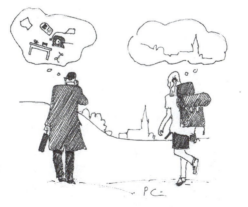

Figure 6.1 Mindlessness and mindfulness

With the possible exception of the latter, the problem with all these strategies is that you do not live in the moment; rather, your mind is populated by the next thing on the 'to do' list or panicking about what you have forgotten to do, or the myriad things you should have done, but have not been able to fit in. Because you are not embodied in and aware of the moment as it passes, but thinking about something else you are, to all intents and purposes, *mindless* of that moment as it unfolds, and consequently are only half awake to the world about you, if indeed you are awake to it at all (see Figure 6.1). Mindfulness is a means of addressing this mindless state *because* it focuses on waking you up to the reality of living in the moment.

Now it is of course common sense that if you are more attuned to the moment and have a more positive outlook on life that you will enjoy it more, feel more balanced and experience a higher state of wellbeing; but the specifics of how you can actually achieve that and what it entails in terms of your everyday life remain rather elusive. If we go back to the description of the Resister (see Figure 5.8), then you can probably safely assume these people are more aware of their personal needs than most, and not only seek out but achieve some personal meaning in life; but are they more awake to, and mindful of, the moment? Not necessarily so; after all, knowing what is meaningful to you and adapting your life to achieve it does not automatically mean the busyness of life or pressures from significant others are also reduced (remember how others responded to Arial's choice in Chapter 3). Consequently, it is useful to consider where you actually are in the sense of living in the moment in your own life in the here and now. In order to help you try to explore this and put it into perspective I will first describe how mindfulness works and then look at how you practice it.

HOW DOES MINDFULNESS WORK?

As noted previously, mindfulness is the process of *attending to the immediate moment* in time and place and that means you have to *actively engage* with it, as it is happening. When you do this several things happen. First, you begin to live in the *present moment* as it unfolds in the here and now. Consequently, you are *not* worrying about the future (whether that is the next ten minutes, or tomorrow or next week) or ruminating on the past; rather, you are paying *active attention* to the moment you are actually in and becoming fully aware of that moment with your whole person, that is, physically, emotionally, psychologically, socially, ethically and spiritually (remember our different dimensions of wellbeing in Chapter 1 – see Figure 1.1). This kind of total awareness is the essence of *engagement;* you become attuned to context, fully experience it, and see and feel new things around you, and through this heightened level of awareness can begin to develop a different perspective on everyday situations.

The thought of having to notice the moment may at first seem rather daunting, but once you get the hang of it, it is, in fact, quite the opposite. This is because once you alter your level of perception to *being* present in that moment, you can also experience heightened awareness in terms of your *attention* to and *engagement* in that moment. Because giving attention and engagement is satisfying, you actually *replenish* your psychic (or attention) energy levels, which means you can *replace* personal resources rather than giving them away (Csikszentmihalyi 1990; 1997).

Logically, this might seem wrong, because I am saying that by expending energy you get some back; but the important point is the *type* of energy. *Psychic* energy is 'attention' energy, used to facilitate engagement and flow. Engagement in an activity stimulates interest and involvement; flow is the peak or optimal experience that can be achieved through engagement in something, and when you attain this level of awareness time can slow down or disappear, and you can feel focused, absorbed and fulfilled. You also experience the passing of time in a meaningful way because you are actually embedded in it and live in each moment, moment by moment.

As a result of paying this kind of attention to time, so you begin to notice it happening and subsequently your perception shifts. When time becomes meaningful to you in terms of your own experience in each moment, so you begin to develop a very different sense of how valuable time is to you and, consequently, how you spend it; when time is *your time, your life,* the passage of *your temporal existence* and the essence of *your being,* then you begin to value each moment because it is important to you; when your mantra is to live each moment in life as if it matters, then you do not give time (your life) away quite so easily.

Again, you may be sitting there thinking that this does not make sense: after all, moving to that way of thinking in the busyness of everyday life is hard, if not impossible, because we are already fraught and stressed. Well yes, for many of us that is the situation but, and this is the important point, it is not being focused and *mindful* in our everyday lives that is stressful, but rather the opposite; it is the more automatic, reactive and frequently unconscious or *mindless* state that we commonly adopt in everyday life that causes the problem (see Figure 6.1).

In this state we activate, often unconsciously, the automatic and learned responses to everyday stimuli. These reactions are roused by the amygdala (see Figure 4.1) and utilize negative thought patterns and disparaging evaluations. This drains the psychic, psychological and emotional energy reserves we have, and erodes our everyday sense of balance and wellbeing.

Mindfulness as a technique addresses this by enhancing our state of awareness or wakefulness in each and every moment in all everyday activities, and consequently can facilitate a more harmonious and balanced approach to life. It serves to fortify our energy levels in all dimensions of wellbeing to support a sustainable and resilient state of health through life balance.

HOW DO YOU PRACTICE MINDFULNESS?

As I touched on in the introduction to this chapter, in order to be mindful you have to engender a state of thinking and way of being in the world that is marked by the three key principles of *intention, attention* and *attitude,* and these require you to actively engage with the process if you want to effectively use the techniques.

Intention is about you *wanting* to do something, in this context, having the conscious direction and purpose or motivation and *intention* to be mindful, to seek wisdom, kindness and wellbeing in everyday life (Brown and Ryan 2003). This requires continued practice, because the normal state of mindlessness will always prevail unless you make the effort to change it; thus you need the ability to pay active and sustained *attention* to the moment. Only through this directed noticing of what is going on around you in each and every moment can you can perceive and experience things happening in the here and now, as they unfold, and consequently generate mindfulness. Finally, *attitude* is about the qualities you personify and how you approach everyday life; it is about embodying a *positive attitude* toward yourself, others, and all living things, animate or otherwise, to facilitate a more harmonious, interconnected and *ecological* approach to everyday life. The phrase *loving kindness* is sometime used to describe this quality (see Figure 6.2).

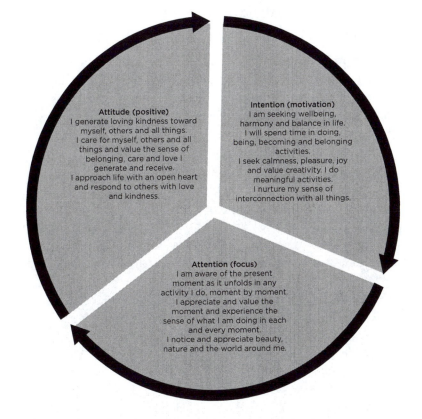

Figure 6.2 Intention, attention, attitude

The skills of mindfulness can be cultivated through formal meditation practice, in which participants sit quietly while directing their attention in specific ways (Kabat-Zinn 1990) and/or through a more informal process of intentionally being aware in each and every moment of the day. This includes paying attention to and experiencing (engaging with) the seemingly mundane activities of everyday life, such as bathing, walking, washing the dishes, eating or working and requires that you begin to *mindfully engage* in these routine tasks. By using this kind of awareness to focus on being fully present and self-aware in each and every moment in each and every activity, whether it is in a *doing, being, belonging or becoming* type, so we can begin to challenge the pervasive state of mindless 'doing' that dominates in modern Western cultures. This means we have to stop clock-watching and rather live *in* time, moment by moment.

MOVING FROM CLOCK-WATCHING
TO LIVING IN THE PRESENT MOMENT

We will talk about time in more detail in the next chapter, but I do want to spend some time thinking about it here. In everyday thinking, time tends to be conceptualized in terms of the macro concept of time. This kind of thinking assumes time is linear, flowing inexorably along a continuum from the past to the present and then on to a future point; this is how we have made sense of our world.

This type of time frame tends to be goal-directed, that is, aiming toward something, and certainly in Western economies we have a *performance orientation*: continually aiming toward growth or productivity. This means that at an individual level we worry about the future, invariably populating our minds with anxieties about performance, fears and insecurities, or we can be ruminating about things that *have*, or indeed *have not*, happened, so in essence are stuck in the past.

Alternatively, micro thinking focuses on the present moment, in terms of the moment to moment passage of time, and it is enacted and embodied in the *here and now*. In this time frame the question or mantra for individuals is, 'Am I really seeing and am I really present in the moment?' (Davidson 2010, p.114).

Whilst the micro view challenges the mindless state of macro thinking, shifting to the micro time frame is not easy: it must be practiced with intention, attention and a positive attitude, which means you have to *want to* attend to and be aware of your connectedness to the present moment in terms of the self and those around you.

Core characteristics of this state have been described as open or receptive awareness and regular or sustained consciousness in ongoing everyday events and happenings (Brown and Ryan 2003). Examples might be that when talking to someone, you are fully aware of the emotional context, and the perception of time may feel elongated or even suspended. I have often experienced this feeling working as a counselor and therapist with clients. In that moment I am fully attuned to the individual and my responses to that individual; I am not ruminating (thinking back) on an argument with my partner, writing my shopping list or worrying about the meeting that is following (future events); rather, I am fully present in the moment.

By centering your attention and whole self in the moment, so you become aware of how you are part of that moment and your related co-evolving and co-production with everything around you; thus you begin to develop a sense of doing, being, belonging and becoming in the moment and your interconnectedness to others and your larger ecosystems.

STEP CHANGES TOWARD BECOMING MORE MINDFUL

Here I just want to run through a simple step change process you can use to begin to practice mindfulness.

STEP ONE: OPEN YOUR MIND

Step one is to open the door to the possibility that mindfulness might just work for you. If you are a therapist reading this chapter then you will know that the first step to achieving personal change is recognizing that you *need* to change; the second is really *wanting* to change (that is the *intention*) and the third is actually *doing* something about it.

This is a particularly important concern in mindfulness practice because intention, attention and attitude require a *positive approach, conscious effort* and a state of *acceptance* to work effectively. Consequently, if you are thinking that mindfulness is a load of rubbish and it is a waste of time, then it is more than likely that it is going to work out just that way for you and, subsequently, you will not benefit from the practice.

To that, I can only say try to open your mind to the possibility that it might conceivably work, and challenge your everyday attitudes and perceptions. In our over-busy and pressured lives, or indeed our mundane, mind-numbing ones, a change in thinking and attitude to achieve a little more awareness of our 'self' in each and every moment could go a long way to enhancing a personal sense of wellbeing. As Langer notes:

> Life consists only of moments, nothing more than that. So if you make the moment matter, it all matters. You can be mindful; you can be mindless. You can win; you can lose. The worst case is to be mindless and lose. So when you're doing anything, be mindful, notice new things, make it meaningful to you, and you'll prosper. (2014, final paragraph)

A positive attitude to life sustains meaningful existence and purpose; it is a tool of resilience in times of adversity. It is not that people with positive attitudes never experience negative affect, but rather that negative affect does not persist (Davidson 2000). Consequently, a move to a more positive perspective can enhance life balance and wellbeing. Look again at the statements in Figure 6.2. These are my own in terms of life balance and may not resonate with you in a meaningful way, so write your own down, but then make sure you begin to live it, however small the initial moves might be; it is worth it because from small moves, big things grow.

STEP TWO: BEING PRESENT IN THE MOMENT

Learning techniques to be mindful is not easy. Much of our day is spent in *mindlessness*, where little attention is given to the present moment. As I have discussed in some detail in previous chapters, life imbalance is often experienced as a frantic juggling of multiple tasks and a paramount concern is completing one task, whilst worrying about the next, or indeed the previous one. This means that you do not engage in or appreciate the fullness of the task in hand. Step two is to address just this lack of awareness and develop your sense of being in the moment; this applies to whatever kind of activity you are enacting, whether that be a doing, being, becoming or belonging pursuit.

Having this kind of awareness of time and place as you carry out or participate in an activity is not how we normally enact our everyday doing. Think about it. Where are you now? How does your body feel in its position in space and what sensations is your body experiencing? How are you feeling emotionally and what are you aware of in your 'sense-scape' if you like? There is no doubt that it is hard to center your 'self' and become aware of your 'self' in place at any one moment, but this is what mindfulness practice tries to convey: the importance of the awareness of being fully present in the moment, and this is what you must learn to pay attention to.

According to Tolle (2005), to do this you need to focus on your inner energy field and become aware of the stillness within you. When focusing inwardly on the body and your inner consciousness, so you can expand the sense of 'being' (existing) in your own body and, through this experience, develop your sense of your 'body-scape' or 'inner-scape'.

This, suggests Tolle (2005), is a doorway to enhancing creative thought because, in essence, you are thinking holistically, with mind, body and consciousness or spirit. The body scan (Box 6.1) is a useful technique to develop awareness of how you are feeling in time, space and place and to become attuned to your bodily sensations. The technique asks you to listen with your whole self, your body and your sensations, as well as with your mind. See if you can feel the energy field in your body as you listen, and allow yourself to feel and come to know your 'inner-scape'. It is coming to know your body and sense 'scapes' inside and out that will allow you to perceive your 'self' in time, place and space.

Box 6.1 *The mindful body scan meditation*

Sit or lie down in a comfortable place and fully relax your body. Let your breathing slow down, and breathe deeply through the NOSE. Feel your abdomen rising and falling and follow the breath from the inhalation through your nose, down into your lungs and then on into your belly.

Follow the breath out in the same way, but starting with the stomach to the lungs, throat, mouth and nose.

Starting with your head, pay attention to your body and notice any tension you're feeling in that area. You might become aware of a feeling of tightness or pain. You might experience a feeling of heat, cold or energy around a certain area. If you do, focus on it for a minute and notice what you are feeling.

If you notice any uncomfortable sensations, focus on them and breathe into them. Notice what happens; the feeling may become more intense at first, then as you continue the body scan meditation and keep your focus, the feeling may dissipate. Keep your awareness on that feeling for a little while, just staying present. Give yourself a little massage in that area if you want to.

Next, move down to your neck, and repeat the body scan meditation steps. Notice if there is any tightness, pain or pressure. Breathe into the areas you notice, and stay with the feelings. Gently massage your neck if you wish. Let your body and mind relax.

Continue this practice with each area of your body, moving from head to toe. Notice how you feel, where you are holding your stress, and what sensations you are experiencing as a result. Breathe, meditate, massage and relax. This can help you release tension in your body now, and be more aware of it in the future so you can release it then, too.

STEP THREE: BE PRESENT IN ALL THAT YOU DO

Another practical technique to develop the skill of living in the moment is to practice being fully present in everyday activities. This can include the rather mundane or routine types of task, like eating, washing up or showering. Have you, for example, ever really been fully present or fully aware of what you are doing with your whole self when you make a cup of tea? I am a lover of tea, so for me this is a great task to start with, but any drink-making or other simple daily activity would do. If you are a chocaholic, try mindfully eating a piece of it. Whatever you choose to experiment with, give yourself ten minutes to really focus on the mindful awareness of the task and approach it with intention (genuine motivation), a positive attitude and your full attention. Box 6.2 works through a suggested tea-making process for you.

Box 6.2 Mindful tea-making

Buy yourself some loose leaf tea if you do not have any, and take down your teapot and dust if off.

Fill the kettle. Turn the tap on and listen to the running water. Be aware of the weight of the kettle changing as you fill it, creating tension in your arm. Breathe deeply and breathe in calm; as you breathe out, let stress leave your body.

Boil the water in the kettle and do not do anything else whilst you are doing that. Focus on the kettle. See it, hear it and sense its presence; it is sharing your space and it is singing, slowly building to a crescendo. Listen to its song.

When the kettle has boiled, pour a small amount of water into the teapot to warm the pot. Place your hands on the teapot and experience the warmth seeping through into your palms and fingers. Smell the hot water – it has a scent all of its own – and sense the heat in your nostrils. Breathe out through your mouth and let your tension go.

Gently swill the water around in the bottom of the teapot and hear its gentle swishing. Pour the warm water out and watch as it tumbles down and disappears into the sink. Listen to the tinkle of the water as it dissipates.

Place a teaspoon or more of the tea leaves into the warmed pot. Smell the aroma of the leaf and study the color. Breathe.

Re-boil the kettle and when it is ready carefully pour the boiling water into the waiting pot. You need about one cup of boiling water to each teaspoon of tea. Watch the steam wafting up and note the aroma of the tea as it infuses.

Stir the brew gently and hear the tinkling of the teaspoon on the china of the pot.

Place the lid on the pot and allow the tea to stand for a minute. Imagine the leaves dancing in the water and notice the smell and feel the calmness.

Pour your tea into your cup and watch the strainer fill; add milk, lemon or sugar to taste. Look at the color of the tea: is it amber, russet, green or black? Smell its aroma; is it earthy, grassy or floral? If you take sugar, smell the sugar as it dissolves; it has a very distinct but almost lucent scent, both there and yet not.

Sip your tea slowly; savour the taste and pay attention to the temperature of the liquid in your mouth. Is it hot, warm, or cool? Notice the taste of the tea and roll it on your tongue. Feel the body of the tea in your mouth and consider its qualities. Is it creamy, full, dry, thin, heavy or light? Swallow and feel the warmth of the liquid infuse you with light.

You might notice that taking the time to enjoy just this one activity enriches all or some of the other activities you do in the rest of your day. This is not because these undertakings have changed, but by apprehending just one activity mindfully, so the quality of your attention to the experience of all others has been enhanced. This is why mindful awareness can enrich life balance, because it changes how you perceive, and subsequently experience, your engagement with life.

Another technique to experiment with in developing this kind of mindful awareness and facilitate a subtle, but meaningful difference in the level of engagement you experience in life, is through changing your established routines and habits. This is a simple and very useful technique to enhance the experience you have in certain tasks in life, even those you do not enjoy.

For example, if you turn back to Box 4.1 in Chapter 4, you will see that the first quote links to established daily routines eroding a sense of balance and wellbeing for the individual concerned. Using mindfulness, this could be addressed by simply taking a different route into work. This change requires attention and higher levels of awareness or engagement to achieve because, as the journey is new and the environment is different, you *have to* plan the route and take more notice. This means you have to pay attention and when you pay attention, you engage in the process. This small change can make a big difference to how you feel, not just in the journey, but in your day because you have experienced engagement. However, key to sustaining your new sense of awareness is to actually experience its unfolding, moment by moment, mindfully: it is only maintaining this level of awareness in the present moment that prevents the re-establishment of routines and habits.

To achieve this on-going practice is, if you like, a process of exercising the mind. First you have to learn to focus on *attending* to the moment in and of itself: the awareness that arises from paying attention on purpose in the present moment and doing this non-judgmentally. The mind, you will find, will go wandering off, seemingly on its own, into your automatic thought cycles, perhaps ruminating or worrying about something or someone; you have to recognize this and gently bring the mind back to its attending to the moment. If there is resistance, it needs to be addressed, and you can do this through continued practice. If you are sitting there thinking that this will not work for you, then remember, small moves *can* make a big difference.

STEP FOUR: SEE THOUGHTS AS THOUGHTS

Step four is becoming aware of your thought streams. This is a very important stage because thoughts are always there, chattering away, often at subliminal levels, which means you have little or no sense of what they are saying to you and, in turn, how you are responding in terms of how you feel or act.

Take a moment to consider, what are you thinking? What thoughts or mental chatter are flowing through your mind right now? Once you get an awareness of your thoughts, you can sense them and feel them but, unlike cognitive therapies, in mindful practice you do not unpick them, rather you observe them non-judgmentally, with idle curiosity, and imagine them drifting past, like clouds in the sky, first into sight and then gently, without concern, out of it.

In mindfulness, thoughts are viewed as mental events, as happenings, which although they can cause physiological and cognitive responses are, in fact, separate from your feelings and bodily sensations. Through practice you gain an awareness of your constant stream of thoughts and become aware of your embedded opinions, values and emotions present in those thoughts, which you can learn to allow to flow through you, without judging them or becoming tangled or immersed in them (Praissman 2008).

In essence, you uncouple the thoughts from the emotional and physical responses, usually in life balance a stress response, and allow yourself to let those thoughts go.

The benefits of the practice of mindfulness are manifold in terms of stress reduction and general wellbeing in life balance, because it offers a tool to review cognitive and emotional schemas in the taken-for-granted social contexts and to recognize them as 'artifacts of our own mindless inattention' (Langer 1992, p.303), which therefore can be restructured to meet personally meaningful requirements.

STEP FIVE: PRACTICE MINDFULNESS

Now obviously you need to practice formal mindfulness techniques if this is to work and there are literally hundreds available on the Internet or to buy on CDs, so I will not run through a full mindfulness practice here. However, I do want to share some simple techniques that you can use on the spot, so to speak, in stressful situations, either in the workplace or other areas of life.

Focus on your breath and breathe

Thich Nhat Hanh (1991a) suggests that everyday situations, which, under normal circumstances you may find frustrating, can be used to practice mindfulness. He suggests, for example, that when you are driving and you get stuck in traffic jams or stop at red traffic lights, you take the opportunity to breathe deeply and smile rather than seeing this as frustrating. This simple technique is something you can start to put into practice today. Use the three breaths technique in Chapter 5 (see Box 5.1) and use Hanh's (1991a, p.33) following mantra to focus your mind: 'Breathing in I calm my body; Breathing out I smile.'

Break the cycle: using mindfulness in stressful situations

By learning and practicing these simple breathing techniques you can use your breathing at key moments to enhance calm, even in on-the-spot stressful situations.

When angry or distressed, breathe and become mindful of that emotion. Hanh suggests another simple mantra to use in these situations; 'Breathing in I know that anger is in me. Breathing out I know that I am my anger.' (1991a, p.57).

When feeling stressed in a particular situation, focus on your breathing and use one of the mantras above, silently if you cannot leave the room or situation. If you can withdraw or take time out, try finding a quiet place, the toilet if necessary, and use the one-minute meditation practice (Box 6.3) to center yourself and induce calm. You can extend this into a longer practice by just breathing slowly and deeply *without* counting the breath in a quiet place, and attend to the feelings within with that non-judgmental idle curiosity I mentioned earlier.

You can do both these kinds of meditation any time and any place, but for best effect walk or sit outside, and if possible be in touch with nature. You can also try out mindful walking and smile at people as you pass. Practicing simple step changes like this in your everyday life will enhance how you feel about yourself and your sense of balance and harmony in life.

> **Box 6.3 One minute mindfulness meditation**
> The first stage in doing this meditation is to count how many breaths you take in one minute. You can do this by either timing yourself or getting someone to time it for you. If you are doing it for yourself, set an alarm and do not clock-watch as this just makes you focus on, or worry about, when the minute will be up. That will not help you relax. Once you have your minute minder prepared, before you start to count it down you need to prepare: make sure you are sitting somewhere comfortable and where you feel safe and calm; place your feet on the floor and make sure you are supported and will not be disturbed; let yourself breathe gently; focus on your breath and get a sense of the breath flowing in and out of your body. Once you feel centered, then start the minute minder and gently focus on your breathing; begin to count the number of breaths you complete in one minute.

Do this by counting as follows: breathe in, then breathe out and count one; breathe in, then breathe out and count two. Repeat this process until your minute is called and then breathe normally, but ensure you remember the number of completed breaths in your one-minute cycle.

The amount of breaths you complete in a minute is unique to you; there is no right or wrong and no element of competition; your number is what it is; no more, no less.

The purpose of the exercise is that you can now carry it with you and practice any time, any place, anywhere a simple one-minute mindful meditation. It can be used prior to a difficult meeting or phone call, following an upsetting event or indeed any time you just need to review, re-balance and re-center. Practice it as often as you can every day.

Adapted from Chakalson 2011.

CONCLUSION: MINDFULNESS AND LIFE IMBALANCE

Mindfulness had become a very popular topic in the media and health and wellbeing literature. Its influence on finding a sense of wellbeing has been focused on seeking psychological, emotional/subjective and, through that, physical, social, ethical and spiritual heath; but, if you think about it, living life in a more mindful way, that specifically emphasizes achieving self-awareness in each and every moment of the activities you do every day, must promote a greater sense of awareness in terms of how you spend your time and energy in everyday life and, consequently, how you use that time and energy to manage your life balance.

Mindfulness, however, is much more than a barometer of how you spend time and energy. First, it can also help by supporting you to become aware of the repetitive patterns you instigate automatically in your daily doings, and second, by making you aware of them, assist, in you being able to extricate yourself from them. By fostering a greater sense of self-awareness about how you live your life, mindfulness can create the opportunity to explore different ways of doing things that could be more congruent with your personal choice, needs and values, namely, who you really are and what you truly find meaningful in life; this will, of course, enhance your sense of self-identity and consequently wellbeing. In essence, by becoming aware of who you are in life activities, so mindfulness can enhance the recognition of one's needs and facilitate a choice of activities across the dimensions of doing, being, becoming and belonging that match your personal interests, values and needs, and consequently help identify those that are meaningful to you.

Interestingly, mindfulness can also assist in engendering a personal sense of autonomy about how you approach activities you find *less* meaningful because, by focusing on them in the moment-by-moment passage of time, so you can become fully aware of the activity and subsequently *engage* with it. This provides the opportunity to think creatively about how you can meet at least some of your needs and wants in *dissatisfying* occupations. In this sense, being mindful allows you to explore different possibilities and potentialities that foster the opportunity for creative engagement in any and all daily activities, including those that you may not find fulfilling. As Easwaran (2008 p.127) says, 'Refrain from doing more than one thing at a time… When you study, give yourself completely to your books. When you go to a movie, concentrate completely on that.'

By enhancing clarity and focus to activities, so mindfulness can add vividness to everyday experience, even in the most mundane of tasks, and consequently can contribute to personal satisfaction and life balance in a very direct way, therefore influencing health and wellbeing.

CHAPTER 7
MEANING AND TIME

INTRODUCTION

This chapter will argue that if we exchange time for meaning, as opposed to money and productivity, then we can establish a *meaning orientation* as opposed to a *performance orientation* in our lives.

I will start by defining what we understand by meaning and time in most Western economies, and then explore ideas about how we can re-orient the use of our time for activities that are personally meaningful to us as individuals.

It is important to note at this juncture, that to this point in the book I have talked about seeking out meaningful activity because it is something that is personally affirming and fulfilling in some way and, consequently, can facilitate a *positive* experience that enables more personal congruence and satisfaction, which, in turn, enhances the quality of life balance.

Now it is of course true that if you enjoy something and it is personally affirming and fulfilling, then you will gain satisfaction from it; but it is also true that some activities are meaningful in the sense of being significant or important for quite the opposite reasons. For example, going to the dentist may be significant because you hate it, and paid work may be meaningful to you because it is associated with high levels of stress. Some of the stories shared by the occupational therapists in this book give insight into this: for many the meanings associated with work, whether paid or unpaid, were stressful, conflictual, anxiety-provoking and deconstructive, and certainly not personally affirming, fulfilling and balancing.

These work activities were, however, viewed as *purposive*, whether it was keeping the house clean and tidy, paying the mortgage, feeding the family or bestowing a sense of identity or role in life; it was something that served a function and was *necessary* to do. This would suggest that when events or activities are enforced on you, socially scripted or defined by others as purposive, then the meaning you derive from that experience can be quite negative *because* the choice to participate in it is expected, whether or not the activity is personally affirming and fulfilling. This is because your sense of personal autonomy over what you do is subsumed by a stronger external locus of control.

These points about the different dimensions of meaning are important to bear in mind as we progress through the book because finding out what is really meaningful to you *personally*, separate from things that are socially scripted or enforced on you, and spending time doing that, is an essential element of living a fulfilling and satisfying life. These types of activities are *autotelic*, that is, they are those we do *for their own sake* 'because to experience it is the main goal' (Csikszentmihalyi 1997, p.117). It is these specific types of *personally meaningful* activities that are both *identity affirming* and *individually fulfilling*, that nourish and enrich our lives and sustain our wellbeing.

Nevertheless, ironically, it is these, of all our activities, that are the most often overlooked or put aside, compromised to use time and energy resources for the *necessary* and obligatory paid and unpaid tasks of life. The loss of these personally fulfilling activities is one of the greatest forfeits we experience in our over-busy lives, because it promotes a lack of meaning and personal fulfillment and it is this void, of all things, that creates the sense of hollowness we carry in our overburdened and imbalanced lives.

In this book I suggest we have to address this, and move from our present performance orientation to a meaning one. This of course is no easy fix and requires change at socio-cultural-political levels, but sticking with our small moves theory of change, I will focus on what we, as people, both individually and collectively, can do to make a difference.

MOVING FROM A PERFORMANCE TO MEANING ORIENTATION

So how then do we move from a performance orientation to meaning one? First, to reiterate, we have to understand that *meaning* in this context, is about your personal drive to find a sense of fulfillment in life. This is not only about purpose, but about what is most important to you, gives you a sense of engagement and satisfaction in life and what enhances your sense of identity, not just in terms of role and function, but in terms of personal *coherence*, or *congruence*: an integrated sense of who you are in life and who you *want* to become.

Clearly this does not suggest a static state, but rather a dynamic one in which we, as individual people, seek to re-orient ourselves toward the meaning of our lives as we interact with our environment and nature. This is exactly what occupational therapists do in order to foster mental and physical health and wellbeing: they facilitate their clients to seek out and find the meaning in their lives and, crucially, to live it in harmony with the rest of life's occupations.

In neoliberal, individualized societies, our search for meaning can be sublimated explicitly into making money, gaining power or seeking obligation, because these can artificially fill the void made for personal meaning and, consequently, detract from the need to seek out and find your actual, personally fulfilling activities.

This happens because money and power are the socially acceptable measures of success and fuel a sense of identity in terms of the 'ought' self, in terms of fitting in and a performance orientation. This provides the means for consumerism and personal security, but it can also lead to overwork, over-busyness, stress, pressure, anxiety and depression. So why do we fall into this trap?

Frankl (2004, p.111) has suggested that people live in an 'existential vacuum', a mindless state marked by a lack of awareness of what is *really* wanted out of life. Consequently, we oscillate between doing what others do (conformism) or what others *want* us to do (remember the ought self? See Figure 5.1). The ultimate outcome of this is chronic stress marked by a state of exhaustion and burnout, or a lack of engagement and rust-out (see Figure 4.5).

Now Frankl (2004, p.115) has a very clear view of where individual meaning or fulfillment lies, and whilst he sees it very much as part of having personal choice in life, he also believes it is about giving to others and 'being' in the world as an active participant, appreciating beauty and nature and creating a work or doing a deed that can be appreciated by others. Accordingly, a meaningful life is not just a selfish desire and an individualized need, but located in a sense of *belonging* with others, *being* in the world, *doing* positive action and *becoming* all that you can be, as well as having the active will or intention to do this.

In this sense, a meaning orientation is found in a complex dance of doing, being, becoming and belonging activities, chosen to facilitate fulfillment in self and others, all wrapped up in the integrated networks of the social and natural worlds (the one we have created and the one that *is*, and which we rely on for life).

Clearly then, seeking a sense of meaning resonates with the concept of balance in doing, being, becoming and belonging activities and mindfulness (see Chapter 6), requiring the will or *intention* on our behalf to achieve it and having a positive attitude and approach; but it is also about finding meaning *in time*, in order to re-orient the use of time to seek meaning.

As I mentioned in Chapter 6, one way to experience meaning in occupation is to facilitate *engagement* or *re-engagement* in certain life activities by focusing our *attention* or *'psychic energy'* onto them (Csikszentmihalyi 1997). This means we have to learn to slow down time through the process of experiencing activity moment by moment. You will recall that I spoke about this 'micro' concept of time in Chapter 6. But the question is, how can we actually enact the exchange of time for meaning instead of money in our everyday lives?

WHAT IS TIME?

In Western cultures time is considered to be *linear* and *sequential*. This is the notion of Newtonian time that most of us know and love: the tick tock of the clock on the mantelpiece that measures the minutes and hours of the day as they pass by and shapes how we spend our time. This kind of time is used to measure the effectiveness of what we achieve every day, and is frequently exchanged for money.

For the paid employee, how much we actively do in the workplace in the time we are being paid for becomes important because we have to spend our time to the best advantage of the organization. This means we are often pressured to do more with fewer resources and it is that measure of time as money that creates the relentless *performance orientation* we discussed in Chapter 2.

WHY DO WE MEASURE TIME IN THIS WAY?

Because we view time as money we ascribe it with *significant value*. This has a couple of negative consequences in terms of a meaningful life balance. First, *face time* or presenteeism in terms of the amount of time we spend doing paid work is measured, because that is equated with productivity in paid work. As a result, cultures that see time as money have a strong *work ethic* and use the principles of capitalism, that is, they see the human worker as a resource in their economic policies.

This kind of thinking about time leads to the imposition of *bureaucracy* and *power structures* in both the workplace and wider society because time has to be managed and controlled in order to be 'spent' in the most economically sound and effective way. This is a problem for life balance because it is an approach that generates conflicts between paid work and the rest of life, that is, it actually crafts work–life imbalance and devalues unpaid work and any other activities, including the personally meaningful ones that do not generate money or growth. This places those who do not participate in paid work for whatever reasons, as subordinate citizens to those who do, and promotes a secondary drive to fill time fruitfully to achieve a sense of self-worth and socially defined purpose or value, which means, in essence, that we create over-busyness.

This has a twofold effect. First, as people become busier and busier, so time is experienced as *speeded-up*; time feels *fragmented* and there is no time to reflect, think or plan, which means no time to be or become. Second, the space for 'doing' activities in any one day becomes *squeezed* as more and more is packed into every minute of the day. As I have previously noted, in this kind of life, time for other pursuits, including those that are personally meaningful in a fulfilling sense, can be lost and this can lead to a sense of meaninglessness in life, a lack of engagement and ultimately burnout and rust-out (see Chapter 4).

Of course, many people do find paid work meets not only their practical needs and social standing (so is purposive) but is also personally meaningful to them (fulfilling) and enjoyable. If that is the case then this is a bonus; but variety in everyday activities is the spice of life and unpins growth in multiple areas of wellbeing (remember the spiritual and ethical dimensions for example?); so a unilateral focus on one activity, even if it is a meaningful one, can lead to obsession, and this is not healthy.

As a recovering workaholic, I am readily aware that spiritual, psychological and emotional/subjective dimensions of wellbeing all suffered terribly in my former life and I was eventually diminished as a person because of it. Moreover, pouring all my psychic energy (attention) into paid work left other aspects of my life bereft of it. How many interests could I have developed, how many more experiences could I have shared and how much more rounded a person would I have become if I had distributed that energy out just a little more equitably?

Sadly, because of the spread of global capitalism, this notion of time as money is becoming commonplace across different cultures and the consequences in terms of wellbeing are proliferating. So how can we address this?

FINDING MEANING IN TIME

Some cultures have a different view of time and consider it more as a *continuum* or *cycle* rather than a linear construct. This concept of time incorporates the circadian or the natural rhythms of time, for example night and day, the changing seasons and the biological cycles of time. The latter are the physiological requirements we all have such as eating, sleeping, resting and toileting.

There is a greater sense of constancy in this sense of time, and its cyclical nature continues whether we stop to perceive it or not. In this kind of approach, time is viewed as fluid, amorphous and consequently creates fewer borders and boundaries between different activities and life domains than the linear constructs of time. Subsequently, the notion of work–life imbalance is not so prominent in cultures working on this time frame, and using time and energy for relationships and meaningful pursuits can be more prominent.

THE RELATIONAL CONCEPT OF TIME

In the relational concept of time, time is viewed as a conduit, or tool that we use to build relationships with significant others and the social and natural environments. Time banking is one form of this notion of time and focuses on investing in emotional connections, like family, friendships, caring and social and community networks by exchanging time for mutual care not for financial gain (Kimmel 2009). Ironically, an effective market economy is actually dependent on sustainable relational contexts, but this is commonly overlooked in performance-oriented cultures (e.g. see the ideas of Sevenhuijsen in Chapter 2 and Kittay in Chapter 3). Another frequently overlooked relationship in a performance-oriented culture is our connection to the natural world. As a result of this loss, we abuse the planet for gain and profit, exchanging wealth for health without a second thought to the consequences.

This again brings us back to the crux of the problem: the time/money interface creating work–life imbalance not only challenges the time and energy of the individual, and subsequently erodes his or her wellbeing, but also impacts on the quality of their family relationships, and their ability to have time and energy to build and sustain social and community networks and ties and to experience the health benefits of the natural world.

TIME AS MEANING

This flows smoothly into the context of time as an experience or measure of meaning. When time is measured by personal meaning it becomes subjective and is frequently experienced as an event or happening in the here and now: 'people do not so much think real time but actually live it sensuously, qualitatively' (Urry 1995, p.6). Because it is a sense of time in the present moment, it has a micro as opposed to a macro temporal quality. You may recall I touched on these notions of time in Chapter 6, where we talked about how we shift to the micro time frame through the use of mindfulness, namely, seeing and attending to the present moment and recognizing and interacting with our connectedness to it, the self and those around us.

When considered in this way, time becomes pertinent to an experience; in essence, it is the subjective feeling about an activity or an event as it unfolds that becomes relevant.

PRACTICAL TECHNIQUES TO PROMOTE A MEANING ORIENTATION

When time is about meaning and not money it accommodates *all* activities in life that have personal meaning. It is not about paid or unpaid work, but about you and what *you* find engaging, specifically those activities you find fulfilling for their own sake. The first step to achieve this is to see time as meaning and, as such, invest in your time wisely: focus on the most important things in both your working and non-working life domains and prioritize them. How do you do this? Well there are a couple of useful techniques.

CONSIDER: WHAT DO YOU REALLY ENJOY DOING WITH YOUR TIME?

In order to answer the question, what do you really enjoy doing, you need to explore and experience different activities to find out. When you know what it is you really enjoy and is meaningful to you, you need to make the time and energy to do it. If you can achieve this then you will have some variety in life; you will not just do work and domestic tasks or other obligations and responsibilities you have to complete to be considered a valued member of society, but experience enjoyment, love and kindness for self and others (see Box 7.1).

Finally, remember that spending time in the natural world is healing, and if you can re-establish your sense of belonging to the planet you will gain one of the greatest sources of harmony and strength for personal resilience that you can possibly access; so use it. This means you have to make space for *being* time and engage with it: making the time to sit and think, to appreciate, and be in and of the natural environment, and just to 'be' or exist in the world. This will harness your spiritual wellbeing as well as your sense of place and belonging to the planet and that will really facilitate your sense of balance in life, because this, of all meaningful pursuits, is the most marginalized in Western life.

> **Box 7.1 What is really important to me**
> Ask yourself, what do you *really* find fulfilling in your life? What is really important to you and what really reflects who you are or want to be?
>
> Try and list six key values and personally meaningful activities and then review these using the following questions.
>
> - Reflect on what your values and personally meaningful activities actually are.
> - Consider whether your values and personally meaningful activities reflect what you really want to achieve or believe is meaningful to you in your life.
> - Consider whether your values and personally meaningful activities reflect how you are living your life now.
> - If not, what changes could be made by you to adapt the life you are living in order to move toward those values and personally meaningful activities?

- Consider how you could readjust your present life balance to accommodate more time and energy to achieve your values and personally meaningful activities.
- Consider how your values and personally meaningful activities impact on the needs of significant others in your life.
- Consider what your values and personally meaningful activities give back to the community and the planet to which you are connected.

HOW DO YOU SPEND YOUR TIME?

Having identified what is important to you, look at the bigger picture and review how you are *actually* spending your time. Whether you are employed, unemployed, not in paid employment or retired, this can be a very useful activity for you to complete.

When you realize your life is out of balance, one of the first things to identify is your total responsibility burden. Ransome (2008) has defined the total responsibility burden as amalgamation of 'necessary labor', that is, the paid and non-paid obligatory tasks carried out in life, and 'recreational labor' or the 'community activities, self-care, leisure, pleasure, enjoyment' occupations you participate in (p.68).

When you start to look at how you prioritize all your everyday tasks, things can start to look a little more complicated. Think of it like this. In the seven days of a week there are 168 hours. How do you spend them? Keep a diary or notebook to record this for an average week. The pie diagram in Figure 7.1 represents a simplified time chart for a particular individual, who for purposes of confidentiality I shall call Lily. When she completed her use of time over an average working week it looked like the scenario in Figure 7.1.

As can be clearly seen, paid work predominated (68 hours = 40%), domestic chores (unpaid work) added another 20 hours (12%) and caring and family commitments another 20 hours (12%) making the total necessary labor up to a total of 108 hours in an average week. The rest of her life activities, including sleep (49 hours = 29%; leisure time: 6 hours = 4%; social: 5 hours = 3%), took a second place to doing these obligatory tasks in terms of time use.

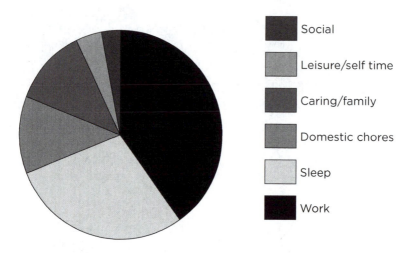

Figure 7.1 Lily's hours spent in average week

Lily lived with a partner and had one older child living at home. She was very stressed and was beginning to experience mild panic attacks in relation to certain work situations. Although she was aware her life was imbalanced and really wanted to change things, she had no idea where to start and was stunned to see how much time she was actually spending on paid and unpaid work tasks. The obvious question to ask Lily then, was why did necessary work take up such a large part of her week?

Why did Lily do so much?

Well, first of all, Lily relished her paid job and this was a very valued and important activity for her; it had *purpose* and *meaning* for her and it was wrapped up with her self-esteem and self-identity: it made her feel good about herself. Second, she worked full-time and *wanted* to do this, but she did feel dissatisfied with what she described as 'constant firefighting' in the workplace rather than a sense of effective completion of tasks. She also described little, if any, control over her own workload, which she felt was jammed to overflowing, causing the constant need to bring work home in order to keep on top of it.

It is important to note that included in her workplace hours was the time taken to travel from home to work and back again. She was keen to point out that she had *chosen* to live some distance from her workplace, but did report that whilst she was, in fact, a reasonably short distance away, she did take some time to traverse the distance in the traditional commuter hours because of traffic (well over an hour) and public transport was poor, preventing an alternative option.

However, whatever rationalizations she came up with to explain why she spent so much time in paid work, she maintained a sense that there was no autonomy or self-determination over her working time and that something was missing in her life. She was not happy and she did feel life could be a little more balanced and fulfilling.

Work at home

At home Lily did the bulk of the housework and caring; indeed 24 per cent of her time was spent doing just that. Her husband certainly helped, but when he reviewed his hours he did not carry an equitable load and his paid working hours were also, in fact, far fewer; consequently, there was space to increase his load at home and decrease Lily's. Lily's son was in his late teens. He was unemployed and did very little in the house at all. His load needed to be increased substantially if he was to carry his fair share of responsibilities in terms of 'necessary labor'. A rota system was developed for all family members, and domestic and caring tasks were clearly and fairly allocated. Whilst Lily's son was not best pleased by this new regime, he did begin to cook, clean, wash clothes and generally develop his domestic skills. All this helped Lily immensely, but paid work remained a problem in terms of balance. So what could she do there, where power dynamics were less equitable?

DEVELOP A SENSE OF AUTONOMY, NOT CONTROL, OVER YOUR TIME IN PAID WORK

There are a plethora of books offering inventories and time management techniques, all of which offer you the opportunity to manage your time in work better. Whilst it is of no doubt that many of these techniques can open your eyes to seeing how your day is spent in terms of time and energy, the problem is that in recognizing these challenges you may not, in fact, be able to address them because you may not have any power or control over that. Consider for example the experiences in Box 7.2. Here an occupational therapist in a healthcare setting (a) and another in social services (b) had no control or power over how they managed their time (a) or their workloads (b).

> **Box 7.2 Limited control over workloads**
>
> a. 'Wednesday afternoon [managers say] "I need it by tea-time." And you have two home visits booked. And then it's, "I am sorry I can't do it"… [they say] "I need it by teatime. You'll have to get it to me by teatime." And what do you do? You know, you've promised to go out and sort out your patient's problem and take out equipment or whatever. But then, you're told by your manager they need information. And that's often because above them, they want it now. So it's being sort of passed through the system.'
>
> b. 'You have to keep your head above water and find your ways to discriminate really, between what's really important and what might appear to be. So you get very astute at getting the facts. So trying to establish what's factual really, with cases that come in. And urgent cases; that sort of tips the balance. If anything, it's the things that you can't plan for.'

We are all subject to external control in terms of power politics, rules and compliance. In the context of life balance, what we require to overcome this is feeling and experiencing a sense of personal autonomy and empowerment in terms of our own lifestyle balance. Now before I begin to explore this, I think it is worth noting that most theories looking at techniques to manage your time suggest the notion of control as a tool to develop this.

Mancini (2003) for example (2003) suggests a very worthwhile strategy to try to develop a sense of control over time and manage it better is by listing your daily activities on a scale of 1–5, with 1 representing an activity over which you have *no* sense of control and 5, something over which you have *full* control. He proposes, for instance, that your morning alarm call is 5 (full control) and morning traffic is 1 (no control). He then advocates that by beginning with those valued as 4, you can practice taking more control and move these activities into a level 5 (full control) scenario. One can, for example, he suggests, develop control over when you answer the phone. Although he concedes this may be less achievable in a work context than a home one, in essence Mancini advocates we can reposition ourselves as in control of our own time.

Personally I think there is credence in this and that we can learn to manage our time better, but there is also an intriguing paradox. I could, for example, suggest that depending on your circumstances, ignoring the phone may not be an option at all and that the morning alarm clock is set by the boundaries of paid work and the travel time it takes you to get there (see Box 7.3 for examples). Of course the travel to work is, to a certain extent, a matter of choice. You can ask yourself and answer the question 'How far am I prepared to travel to work?' But there are always contextual issues that shape how much control you have over the answer to that question and what you can do in that situation; when you set the alarm is purely dependent on the options or choices available to you. Consequently, the word 'control' is, in one sense, arbitrary as the control frequently lies with externalized forces, and thus it is a word of dominance. An alternative to control is autonomy, which resonates with the notion of an *internal* sense of *empowerment* and locus of control as opposed to that external one.

> ### Box 7.3 Contextual issues that externally shape and control choice
>
> a. 'It's difficult because of how we approach work, sort of, generally as you know in the Western world and having 8 out of 14 waking hours in one place already makes it a little bit imbalanced.'
>
> b. 'So since we moved here, it's now a minimum of 30 minutes for me to get to work. But if I leave any later than 7.55 then it takes me 45 to 50 minutes to get here. So I really have to leave the house at 7.30 in the morning or maybe max 7.45. So 7.45am till about 6 o' clock to 6.30pm I'm out of the house. So I have four waking hours a day for my own time. So... if I get back at 6 o' clock I go to bed at 10; read till 10.30 'cos I'm too tired after and go to sleep by 10.30'.

SET ACHIEVABLE GOALS

Another method commonly presented as a strategy to take control (or more appropriately gain a sense of autonomy) over your time is prioritizing the tasks on your 'to do' list. Perhaps most well-known is the ABCD method, which purports that you categorize your tasks in terms of their *time sensitivity* (Mancini 2003).

In this context those tasks attributed as A are critical in terms of time; B are urgent but not as critical as A; C are important, but can wait; and finally, D are not time-sensitive at all, and could be ignored or delegated.

Perhaps most interestingly, Mancini (2003) argues that it is the D activities, albeit not time driven, that can be surprisingly useful to engender a sense of autonomy, because it is these very activities that may offer solutions for doing things differently, or more effectively, in the workplace. It is these activities that can provide the self-time, reflective time and thinking time, the 'being' activities if you will, and will assist in developing yourself and your sense of autonomy over your own work and life balance. If you consider the message in this book, this idea that accessing these kinds of pursuits will improve your effectiveness in paid work is not so surprising. Indeed, I would posit this technique would be beneficial in *all* life domains, and would be especially valuable for treating the Rushaholic, Busyaholic and Busy Bees. The urgent/important matrix is another example of a tool that has similar uses and applications.

THE URGENT AND IMPORTANT MATRIX

In theory, this technique will also help you to prioritize your time by organizing your tasks in an effective way. Again, although traditionally applied to the paid workplace, I would advocate its usefulness in all life domains. So how do you use it? The first stage is to make a list of the tasks you have to do. Look at your diary and to do list to help you with this. Allocate a number 1–5 against each task to assign its importance, but do this in terms of reaching your *goals and objectives* and *not* its urgency. This is a subtle, but notable, difference from the ABCD model. When you have done this, plot it onto the matrix as shown in Figure 7.2.

Whilst the matrix helps you to physically see how your tasks are prioritized, it can also assist with a visual measure of stress levels. In essence, in order to manage stress levels, the *'not urgent but important'* activities should take up the most of your time and by sound priority management, be kept and completed at this level rather than progressing to 'urgent'. If you have too many *'urgent and important'* tasks then you are at risk of moving into stress and burnout. You have to consider which of these tasks you have left too late to complete (your problem) and those that you could not foresee (as per the examples in Box 7.2) and whether or not *you* should have allocated time for such emergencies.

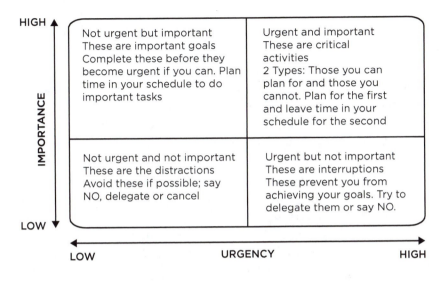

HIGH

IMPORTANCE

LOW

Not urgent but important	Urgent and important
These are important goals Complete these before they become urgent if you can. Plan time in your schedule to do important tasks	These are critical activities 2 Types: Those you can plan for and those you cannot. Plan for the first and leave time in your schedule for the second
Not urgent and not important These are the distractions Avoid these if possible; say NO, delegate or cancel	Urgent but not important These are interruptions These prevent you from achieving your goals. Try to delegate them or say NO.

LOW   URGENCY   HIGH

Figure 7.2 The urgent and important matrix
Adapted from Mindtools (2003).

Looking at Box 7.2, for example, it is possible that those 'urgents' at work (2), if they are a regular occurrence, could be planned for. Alternatively, workloads delegated by managers without warning (1) cannot be, and consequently are far more difficult to manage, as contingencies cannot anticipate such random variables or address the power dynamics and demands for immediate action. In this situation you have to consider how you can achieve a sense of autonomy in terms of time in the workplace, or indeed the home (e.g. Box 7.3b), when the decision-making is externalized. I will return to this in Chapter 8.

Looking at the third and fourth quadrants, if several of your tasks are *urgent but not important*, then think about the nature of those tasks and contemplate whether they are other people's work or, on reflection, are not necessarily essential to either the organization's or your personal goals. Consider the example in point a, Box 7.2. Here, the occupational therapist is responding to pressures from above; is this her work and goal (i.e. part of her role expectations) or is she being delegated a task that should have been completed by her manager or given to someone else? Either way, the short timescale and lack of preparation time has resulted in a conflict scenario and a reactionary, firefighting approach to meet the deadline.

Finally the *'not urgent and not important'* activities can, so the theory goes, be struck off your list completely by, for example, being cancelled or delegated. This is an interesting thought, as one must question what these activities are and how does one assign them with this dual status of not important or not urgent? Does it include email sorting or filing? These are distractions but they *do* need to be done. If it is coffee with colleagues or lunch out of the office, then should these be knocked off the list? If it is a walk in the park, or an opportunity to think or reflect, should this be removed? If your answer to these questions is yes, then perhaps these activities need to be re-evaluated by you and placed in the important but not urgent category. Certainly, some people in my studies did do this and made changes in their everyday lives to accommodate what was important to them outside of the paid and unpaid work domains by making time for activities, which may not have been valued by others, but were meaningful to them. Hence the key lesson is yes, by all means get rid of the unimportant and not urgent tasks that can be delegated or left to others, but do not compromise your meaningful activities; rather, make the time for them *a priority*; these things are too essential to *your* fulfillment and wellbeing in life to be forgotten or ignored.

So how can you do this when external powers and social drivers can prioritize the necessary or obligatory tasks, and paid work is so greedy it takes more than it should? That is a very good question and one I hope to answer in the next chapter, but as an initial step, you need to adjust your own thinking and review your personal meaning orientation.

THE VALUES, CHOICE AND RECONCILIATION CYCLE

Figure 7.6 describes the values, choice and reconciliation cycle. The cycle is really a way of thinking about how you can reconcile meaning in life with the choices available to you in your external environment. I will talk much more about the notion of reconciliation in the next chapter, but here I will work through the cycle with you to identify its use as a technique for gaining a sense of autonomy over your own life balance in order to introduce more personal meaning into your life.

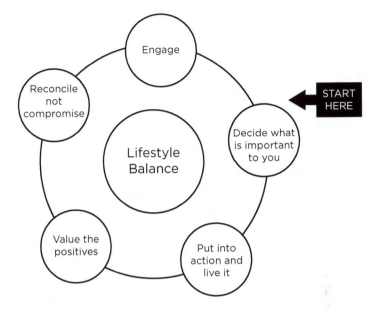

Figure 7.3 The values, choice and reconciliation cycle

Stage 1: Awareness

First, begin at the beginning and decide what is important to you in your everyday life; what activity do you really enjoy doing and how does it give you a sense of meaning? Answering this question is a good start – awareness is not always there and it can be very hard for the individual and the confidante or therapist to help people wake up to the source of meaning in their everyday lives. When you do give it some thought (see Box 7.1), you may find you have many such activities in your life, but initially start with one. You can always repeat the cycle and build more in later.

Stage 2: Intention and will

When you know what it is that you want to make time for, actually make the time to do it. Start small; if it is running, do not plan to run every day but aim for once a week, on a day where pressures are less, for example say a Sunday morning or a Friday evening. This makes it achievable and success leads to satisfaction and greater motivation to make the time and energy to do more of the activity. Remember, small moves can make a difference. The outcome is you will begin to feel more alive, fulfilled and creative in life.

Stage 3: Positive thinking

We talked a great deal in Chapters 5 and 6 about the power of positive thought and in this context you must apply this principle and value the positives; think not that you are only running once a week, but that you *have* achieved it: you *ARE* running once a week and it makes you feel good, so very good. Live in the moment, moment by moment; when you are doing the meaningful activity, *really* enjoy it.

Stage 4: Reconciliation not compromise

The process of reconciliation will be described in more detail in Chapter 8, but I will contextualize it briefly here. To reconcile means to restore friendly relations, or make compatible, whilst compromise, alternatively, means to make concessions. In neoliberalism we are programmed to accept the compromise of our own use of time and energy in terms of personal meaning and consequently wellbeing, in order to meet socio-cultural-political and economic obligations in terms of life balance, and the question has to be why? I have talked about making compromises in terms of meaning in life throughout the book, and elsewhere have coined the term 'occupational compromise' (Clouston 2014, p.514) to capture the nature of this commonly chosen tool for dealing with life's conflicts in terms of time and energy. But what if you could view it differently? What if meaning *was* your priority in life?

Please note here that I am not advocating you should be selfish or narcissistic; these kinds of behaviors are as damaging as compromising your own wellbeing because self-orientation prevents one's search for true meaning in life; 'being human always points, and is directed, to something, or someone other than oneself' (Frankl 2004, p.115). What I am suggesting is that as individuals, in order to tackle the conflicts we presently experience in harmonizing our busy lives with finding time and energy for meaningful activities, we have to find the will, or intention, to re-orient ourselves toward our own unique meaning in life and give it the attention or psychic energy it deserves *because* this is the human being's primary motivational force. This, then, requires a change to our normal thinking and attitude: you have to make the effort to focus on the bits you like doing and believe, however paradoxical this might seem, that by doing this, you will feel the benefit and be *less* stressed. It is the letting go (compromising) of them that is the problem and re-orienting yourself to finding meaning in life is the solution.

Stage 5: Engage

By accomplishing the meaningful activity you will achieve a sense of personal fulfillment, wellbeing and through this, harmony and balance in life. You can further enhance this by focusing your attention (or psychic energy) fully into that activity when you are actively participating in it. This has a twofold outcome. First, you will begin to *engage* in the activity and fully appreciate the experience of it in the moment; second, through this you will begin to experience flow.

Having achieved the first five stages of your values, choice and reconciliation cycle, you should be experiencing a greater sense of balance and consequently harmony, fulfillment and wellbeing in your everyday life. So what now? Well, as the first stage of this cycle suggested, it is time to move on to a second meaningful activity or, if there was only one to achieve, increase the amount you participate in that into your daily repertoire of life. This is of course not easy, but having completed the cycle once, you should feel that it is worth doing and as it makes you feel good, the will, intention and motivation should be there to continue. This process will help you to think about where to focus your attention (psychic energy) and serve to sustain your sense of meaning and purpose in life. In the next chapter I will take this notion of reconciliation a stage further and consider how that could apply at an organizational, relational and wider socio-cultural-political contexts.

CONCLUSION

In practice, in neoliberal economies at least, we compromise our own personal meaning activities to achieve what we feel we should do or what others believe we should do (remember the ought self). Of course, obligations have to be made, not only in terms of safety and security (earning money to live) but also for love and belonging (caring for others); yet, and this is the important point, these are *not* exclusive needs. It is the search for meaning that creates a personal sense of fulfillment in life and this is the lost element of life balance: the one we give away or *compromise* to meet the challenge of our over-busy lives. The answer then must be to incorporate a meaning orientation into your life.

However, there is one word of warning when on this quest: continually ask yourself, are these choices in terms of personal meaning really mine or are they derived from socio-cultural-political values, the expectations of significant others, the power dynamics in the workplace, or are they socially motivated? It is always a question worth thinking about in a work-driven, consumerist society; and remember, time shapes identity and who we are is a reflection of how we spend our time; time use is a measure of what we have done, are doing and will become; time is meaning so use it wisely.

CHAPTER 8
CREATING WELLBEING IN WORKPLACES

INTRODUCTION

In the last couple of chapters I have shared techniques that can help you to balance your life a little more, including reclaiming your autonomy over life balance and re-establishing your personal sense of self by moving toward a meaning orientation in your everyday occupations. These strategies are effective and certainly do enhance the quality of your life balance, but, however courageous you are in fighting the good fight to get meaning back into your life, there remains one big problem: the wider socio-economic-political cultures that create and shape the power dynamics in the workplace, the attitudes and values of significant others, including families, the workplace, and social networks that inveigle themselves into our lives and shape the options and possibilities available to us in our little corner of the world.

So how can we overcome this? Well, in truth, it seems that when it comes to work, paid or otherwise, we do have to make the best of a bad job and make some sort of compromise; even Arial, who was a true freedom fighter, had to do that: she compromised promotion, salary and value in the workplace, and consequently talked about doubting her choices and pondering on the what if's, 'What if I had gone all out and been a career woman? Would my life have been better?'

Now whilst Arial had deliberated on this, she had also, quite unusually, found a solution to her unanswered question by reconciling herself to this loss. By working through the values, choice and reconciliation cycle (Figure 7.3), she had reached a point of personal appeasement and could feel *satisfied* with her choices about paid work and home, however much colleagues in the workplace riled her about it, because she *knew* time at home was really what she wanted. But this sense of personal resolution was not so marked for other occupational therapists, who found they could not reconcile their losses so easily. Jenna for example, *could not* apply for promotion because the organization would not allow her to work part-time in a management position and she *had to* work part-time because she had caring commitments to meet, which could not be outsourced (see Chapter 3).

As workers, we can frequently find ourselves in this sort of situation: organizations are more powerful than individual employees and hold the majority of cards in terms of choice over working hours and pay (remember numerical and temporal flexibility in Chapter 3). Neoliberal labor markets increase this imbalance by promoting individualism and denouncing collective action and unions; eroding long-term contracts and encouraging flexibility; and building power and choice for organizations and rescinding those rights for employees. They thus decrease the responsibilities carried by the employer, but increase those of the employee, making the latter the responsible agent when things do go wrong.

So what if you find yourself in this situation and you want to have some sense of fulfillment or satisfaction in your daily work, paid or otherwise, but the workplace culture, values of significant others or social norms preclude this? Both Jenna and Arial experienced this; they just had different ways of dealing with it because their meaning orientations differed, with Jenna being far more work-centered than Arial.

This chapter will explore these problems and consider how we can address the challenges in our paid and unpaid workplace. There are two interweaving strands to this. First, the chapter considers the notion of *reconciliation* as a tool to achieve balance between work, paid or otherwise, and the rest of life, as opposed to the traditional concept of compromising activities to overcome these conflicts. Second, the chapter will challenge us to re-evaluate how we traditionally view relationships in the workplace, to re-envision them as *relational networks*, where people care for one another and create *meaningful* human interaction.

RECONCILIATION: CHALLENGING THE DILEMMAS OF WORK–LIFE BALANCE

We discussed in some depth in Chapter 2 the dilemmas people can experience in terms of work–life balance when employed in organizations. I am sure that many readers identified with those dilemmas and resonated with the compromises people made to manage them. Here I want to revisit those dilemmas and consider them in the context of the organizational and cultural *reconciliation* model devised by Woolliams and Trompenaars (2013), as opposed to the more traditional approach adopted in the work–life balance *compromise* model.

RECONCILIATION VERSUS COMPROMISE

You will recall from Chapter 7 that to reconcile means to restore friendly relations, or make something compatible, whilst to compromise means to make concessions. This is a subtle, but notable, difference, where harmony (in the former,) rather than loss (in the latter) is achieved. So how can we do this when power dynamics in organizations or local cultures control interactions and indicate otherwise?

The first stage for you is to work through the values, choice and reconciliation cycle I introduced in Chapter 7 (see Figure 7.3), and apply this specifically to the workplace context, because this will help you to identify what you enjoy most about your job.

By doing this you will begin to rekindle an interest in your work and consequently be able to re-engage with it; you may even engender a sense of personal autonomy in the workplace (see Box 8.1).

The values, choice and reconciliation model may engender a sense of personal autonomy over your working life, but as I have discussed in some depth, the problem with achieving satisfaction or fulfillment in work situations is that the workplace power dynamics or pressures can frequently challenge your personal choices and the culture or wider social values may be at odds with your own wishes or beliefs.

Box 8.1 Values, choice and reconciliation cycle in work

STAGE 1: AWARENESS

At work, what activity or aspect of the job do you really enjoy doing? Like in the wider life context, this can be hard to pinpoint but something, however small, will be there. For example, you may be disengaged at work but realize you enjoy the problem-solving aspect of your job; you may be burned out, but remember that once upon a time, you really enjoyed the client contact in your job. You may feel under-valued and apathetic about housework, but remember the sense of satisfaction you get when the house is clean, or that pleasure you experience in ironing when watching a good film. Whatever it is, find it.

STAGE 2: INTENTION AND WILL

Once you have it, know it and do it. If it is something you already do every day (e.g. the problem-solving aspect of your job), then notice when you are actively doing it in your daily work. If it is something carried out less frequently, then just make sure you notice it when you *are* doing it and plan to incorporate more of it into your week. Start small, with achievable goals.

STAGE 3: POSITIVE THINKING

Think not 'I am stressed' or 'disengaged' but 'I *am* seeing clients and enjoying it', 'I love problem-solving and it *is* still here in my daily work' or 'Yes, I do feel pleased when the house is clean and that *is* a job well done.'

STAGE 4: RECONCILE

Do not make compromises because the pressures feel too great or the options limited; rather, remember the good bits in the job: focus on your problem-solving, embrace your time with clients and definitely do the ironing with a good film on. Why not?

STAGE 5: ENGAGE

Finally, engage in those meaningful or enjoyable aspects of your work; be present in the moment as you do them and open yourself to the potential of enjoying work a little more, and even the possibility of experiencing flow. You never know…

These kinds of tensions or dilemmas, born of relations between employee, employer and socio-cultural-political and economic constructs create work–life imbalance and several examples of these were noted in Chapter 2. Woolliams and Trompenaars (2013) argue that these kinds of dilemmas exist in all organizational settings and are multifaceted and complicated by the drive for productivity. This creates conflicts between the needs and wellbeing of the employee and the business process, which is interested in corporate effectiveness; the shareholders, who are interested in shareholder return, hence growth and profit; the clients/customers, who are interested in satisfaction, and the wider society in which the organization is situated, because that, too, will want a contribution, usually of an economic kind. They developed their model of reconciliation to specifically address the ensuing conflict scenarios that occur as a result of these tensions at an organizational level.

THE MODEL OF ORGANIZATIONAL RECONCILIATION

Woolliams and Trompenaars (2013) suggest the first step in their model of reconciliation is to review the conflict in terms of what has to be done to achieve a positive outcome for both parties. To do this, you simplify the conflict situation into a win–win scenario for both sides, using the prefix of 'On the one hand we want to…' and 'On the other hand we want to…' which places the conflict into the outcomes you want for both parties. Using this approach, they have identified ten recurrent dilemmas emerging from a variety of different workplace settings and countries around the world, which they have called the 'golden dilemmas' (Woolliams and Trompenaars 2013, p.11). Table 8.1 illustrates three examples that seem, for me, to be specifically pertinent to the dilemmas that can occur in work–life balance.

To consider how can we use this reconciliation model in the specific examples of work–life conflict raised in the book, I want to work through the examples noted in Chapter 2 and consider how this process could assist in finding solutions. You may recall that the dilemmas I identified in this chapter were: workplace intensification versus employee stress; lack of employee control and choice; a culture of fear and insecurity for employees; resource constraints preventing flexibility for employees; a lack of emotional support and care for employees; a performance versus health and wellbeing culture; and finally, the pressures of self-identity as a valued worker and self-responsibility creating a performance orientation (see Chapter 2). As a first stage I will consider if these resonate with the golden dilemmas noted in Table 8.1.

Table 8.1 Three golden dilemmas of work–life balance

Dilemma	On the one hand	On the other hand
1	**(Employees)** We need to develop our people for their future roles in different ways of working.	**(Business Processes)** We need to become more cost conscious and results-oriented.
2	**(Employees)** We need to empower, motivate and reward our people to work in new ways.	**(Shareholder)** We need to satisfy our shareholders that their investment will remain secure as newer ways of working become the norm.
3	**(Employees)** We need to retain equal opportunities for all existing staff and recognize their differing personal values.	**(Society)** We need to apply some positive discrimination to increase diversity and recognize the new and changing world of work.

Adapted from Woolliams and Trompenaars (2013, p.10).

REVIEWING THE DILEMMAS

At first glance, the first seven dilemmas listed in Chapter 2 have a direct employer versus employee conflict. However, the wider socio-cultural-political and economic influences (in this case neoliberalism) were also evident in all examples, and specifically redolent in the dilemma of a self-identity formed through the notion of valued worker and drive for employee self-responsibility.

Looking at Table 8.1, the first golden dilemma is about the need to achieve organizational productivity AND invest in the needs of the individual worker in terms of new ways of working; this is a classic work–life balance issue and one Woolliams and Trompenaars (2013) believe can be overcome *if* the organization strives to reconcile both in a meaningful and effective way. Several of the dilemmas in Chapter 2 could be classified in this way, which, theoretically at least, means that rather than experiencing a drive for organizational performance over employee health and wellbeing, the dilemmas of intensification causing stress, and resource constraint preventing opportunities for work–life balance, the employee *could* also have benefited, as well as the organization, if the reconciliation approach had been implemented (see Figure 8.1).

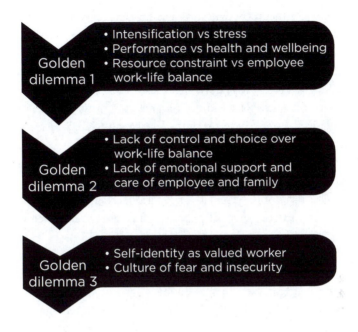

Figure 8.1 The seven work–life balance and three golden dilemmas

Framing the reconciliation approach

So how could we deal with these conflict situations by using reconciliation and not compromise as a solution? Woolliams and Trompenaars (2013) suggest that one technique might be to invest in the staff group to get them to understand how to reduce costs and maintain productivity, so they become part of the solution not the problem. This would certainly impart a sense of greater autonomy for the worker, but in order to create any personal meaning from this, the organization, at the same time, would have to review how it views its staff group and move away from a purely human *resource* perspective to one that values the employees as workplace, family *and* community members. This is much more of a *communitarian* or *collective* stance than the traditional *individualist* approach and consequently challenges neoliberal labor market principles.

This, of course, is not easy; within the organization, it requires a fundamental movement in thinking and a culture that supports a more flexible workplace for employees to meet not only family and caring responsibilities, but their own self-care needs, as well as facilitating community participation and personally meaningful activities. This directly opposes the 'more with less' cultural approach taken in the use of human resources in most neoliberal workplaces, which results in employee personal requirements and meaningful pursuits being compromised.

Golden dilemma 2 (Table 8.1) is about supporting, valuing and empowering staff to work flexibly, feel cared for and supported *and* meet the expectations of stakeholders in the organization. This dilemma resonates with those in Chapter 2 in terms of the *lack of control and choice* employees experienced over workload, time and energy use in the workplace (thus work–life imbalance) and the *lack of emotional support and care* from others in the workplace, which, in terms of the experiences shared, led to compromises in autonomy, self-determination, family health and wellbeing, and limited or absent personally meaningful doing, being, belonging and becoming activities.

Woolliams and Trompenaars (2013) suggest that balancing time at home and having a decent personal life with the need to work longer hours to gain more profits for the shareholders can cause employee work–life imbalance and that this is directly related to a lack of personal integration between *doing* and *being* activities or an overdeveloped performance orientation that does not fit with the individual's personal preferences and choice. Although Woolliams and Trompenaars (2013) do *not* note the compromises of becoming and belonging time and energy clearly evidenced in this book, the reconciliation model does suggest that cultural change to support meeting both stakeholder and employee satisfaction is possible and that this, if achieved, will be a win–win situation, namely, of benefit for both parties – organizational stakeholders and employees. Although no practical suggestions are made in Woolliams and Trompenaars' (2013) paper, for me a more caring and egalitarian approach to flexible working, and a relational approach to cultural values, would have gone some way to attaining this outcome.

The third golden dilemma (Table 8.1) suggests that organizations have to ensure both a person-centered and equitable approach to employees, but also adopt systems that may positively discriminate for organizations in order to maintain productivity in the changing marketplace (e.g. deregulation of markets and numerical working patterns). This resonates with all the ethical dilemmas the occupational therapists were experiencing in their respective workplaces around the notion of the ideal employee and flexible working, but here I will note the two remaining dilemmas from the list in Chapter 2, which are a direct consequence of neoliberal practices: the construct of self-identity and self-worth located in being a paid worker (or over-busyness if not in paid work) and an increased sense of personal responsibility in the workplace, associated with the ensuing culture of insecurity and fear in terms of losing opportunities or perceived value in paid work (see Chapter 2). These two dilemmas are fully enmeshed in the opposition between socio-cultural-political and economic drivers and the needs of the individual worker, so fall straight into the employee versus society paradigm (see Table 8.1).

For Woolliams and Trompenaars (2013) this, like all their dilemmas, can be reconciled by fundamental culture change; but this, of course, is also the stumbling block in terms of this approach: can socio-cultural-political processes transpose their thinking so creatively in terms of economic models to be able to move from notions of growth and productivity to sustainability, from pressure and stress to wellbeing and resilience, and from individualism to relational networks? This is a key question and one I will return to in the next chapter, but here I do want to consider what this kind of culture might look like in the workplace setting if we could make that change.

WHAT MIGHT THIS CULTURAL CHANGE LOOK LIKE IN THE WORKPLACE?

First, the new culture would need to dissolve the division between work and life in order to view it as an integrated whole, where work is enriched by the rest of life and vice versa. Second, people would need to be recognized and valued as products of multiple roles, domains and activities, rather than just work: in essence, appreciated in all their complexities as occupational beings. Third, in order to sustain these perspectives all the domains (family, social, community and natural to mention but a few) and all the activities (including personally meaningful ones) that people participate in, would need to be valued socially and culturally as much as paid work, because, in terms of life balance and human health and wellbeing, all are essential and consequently indivisible.

Using the notion of doing, being, becoming and belonging is a useful construct for achieving this concept of life balance because it embraces complex interactions and embodies a meaning orientation as opposed to a performance one. According to Davidson (2010, p.115) we can support a transition to a meaning orientation in all human settings by seeing and attending to the connections between people, because meaning exists in the complex networks of personal interactions: 'Meaning is born out of the experience of conversation that occurs in the micro-present (living present)... it is individuals and their interactions with each other in the living present that make up an organization.' In this sense it is not just the choice of activity that makes something personally meaningful, but the interaction or the network of others in which that activity takes place. In fact, the organization or domain of work exists only because of the interaction of people. When you think about it, this is, of course, common sense; and yet it is the human element that is most frequently ignored in conventional thinking about work.

RELATIONAL AND ALTRUISTIC VALUES IN THE WORKPLACE

When we feel, react and respond as human beings in action with, and as a result of, others in the same place, then the emotional exchange between us becomes reciprocal and *people*, rather than *task*, become the central context of what we do.

If we approach both the paid and unpaid workplace with this attitude, then the notions of work–life balance that are held within that setting become a product of the relational factors that go on within it; if this can be more caring, then, so the theory goes, the approach and attitude to supporting imbalance, burnout or rust-out can become one of nurture, not blame (Meyerson 2000). In this kind of cultural construct, it is the essence of the relational network in and of itself that becomes integral to the success of the workplace:

> Good work is not just the maintenance of connections – as one is now said to work 'for a living' or 'to support a family' – but the enactment of connections. It is living, and a way of living; it is not support for a family in the sense of an exterior brace or prop, but is one of the forms and acts of love. (Berry 2002 p.133)

So how can we generate this kind of relational network in our workplace culture and our lives? How can we weave respect and egalitarianism into the weft of the web of life balance?

MOVING TO A RELATIONAL CULTURE

Reiter (2007) has argued that if we are to achieve a more caring and altruistic or egalitarian approach to work, then the models of flexibility found in organizational settings need to be viewed from an ethical standpoint and not a performance orientation. She offers four different positions that organizations can adopt in this ethical dimension, and describes these as follows (numbers have been added to assist in identifying the four standpoints):

> A situationist position (1) focuses on a 'fitting' definition of balance for a person depending on his or her personal context. This will include their stakeholders, resources, and desires… The subjectivist definition (2) will be concerned only with the individuals' desires, an 'anything goes' type definition suggesting that as long as they are happy with their [work–life balance], nothing else matters… an absolutist perspective (3) accepts that rules can prescribe a 'right' formula for balance… This contrasts with exceptionists' definitions (4) that are of a utilitarian nature and seek to reflect the greatest good for the greatest number. (Reiter 2007, p.275)

Reiter purports that the situationist perspective is the one that should be adopted in the workplace to achieve an ethical approach to work–life balance, 'because these definitions will involve making optimum choices for each individual' (p.276). As I noted in Chapter 3, she maintains, 'It is employers who facilitate this outcome that will truly be employers of choice' (p.276).

Now this perspective clearly suggests a person-centered focus, where employees' subjective choices and desires are paramount, but it also considers their situational context: the stakeholders and resources available, and thus the wider familial and relational networks inside and outside of paid work, so in essence it assumes a more *communitarian* or *collectivist* stance. By accommodating both concepts, that is, both a person-centered and embedded context, could this approach reconcile the difference in the workplace dilemmas experienced in Chapter 2?

Clearly the workloads and work pressures were a huge problem in terms of stress and work–life imbalance for employees and addressing this could only have helped, but the psychological overlay from feelings related to negative relationships and perceptions of bullying and professional disenfranchisement also required addressing, and a more mindful, empathic and collective, relationally focused approach would have assisted in building bridges and a spirit of community and belonging. Meyerson (2000, p.180) has suggested that if workplace cultures are to provide support for life balance, then they have to sustain a culture that 'could legitimate and enable the emergence of communities that care for their members and provide conditions for human connection and autonomy.' It is also of no doubt that the principles of understanding the value of others in the family, the social/community domains and wider culture and creating, as part of those networks, a caring and nurturing environment can only support a more egalitarian and altruistic approach to life balance. As Putman (2000, p.21) put it, 'A society characterized by generalized reciprocity is more efficient than a distrustful society and as such trustworthiness lubricates social life'.

However, we all know that for strategies to be effective at these multiple levels necessitates not only support within the workplace setting and its embedded cultures, but at wider socio-cultural-political and economic levels, meaning that this kind of move involves fundamental structural change. This requires working together to achieve a caring, cooperative and emotionally astute community of action. In such a complex web, what can we, as individuals, do? We can make small moves.

THINK ABOUT RELATIONSHIPS AND NURTURE PEOPLE IN THE WORKPLACE

The organization and its culture do not exist separately from the people who are in the organization. As Mintzberg, Ahlstrand and Lampel (1998, p.264) cogently remarked: 'culture knits a collection of individuals into an integrated entity called organization.' What this suggests in terms of work–life balance is that the attitudes held within the organization are a product of all of the relational factors that go on within that organization: the organization is a product of both people and environmental forces and consequently is a creation of the economic, political and social structures of which it is a part.

The organizations I studied were coercive in their use of power and used fear, namely, threats of job losses or being passed over for promotion, as the subconscious tool of behavior management. You, as an individual, cannot change these kinds of power lever on your own, but you can change how you enact them and what you do as an individual in the workplace to support and create a more person-centered, emotional and supportive link with others. This again is the small move theory: you make a change and others, especially the like-minded, will also benefit.

If [you] can help those people who already share certain beliefs and dreams sing their songs a little clearer, a little more confidently...

they will take that song back to their networks… We gain courage from knowing we're part of choir. We sing better when we know we're not alone. (Wheatley 1999, pp.151–152)

Here are some simple techniques you could put in place to help you and your choirs sing in harmony:

Be genuine and honest with one another

- When you are in your workplace, ask people how they feel and *listen*: really *hear* them and then *respond* to what they have said. When you *genuinely* value others that will be reflected back.

- Give *feedback*. Tell people when they do something well and offer support when things do not go too well. Be *open* and *honest* when you feel stressed and *genuinely* listen to others when they speak to you about their difficulties.

- Within your teams, look at systems or strategies that you can put into place to *support* and *accept* one another.

- As mentioned in previous chapters, *share* pressures and workloads. Do not use this as a tool to *promote* and *escalate* pressure, for example, the 'I am doing more than you and therefore you are not doing enough or carrying your fair share' scenario. The total responsibility burden described in Chapter 7 is a method to do just this in the non-paid home domain and any positive changes there will help you function better in paid work too. Remember, work and home domains exist within you and consequently, you are one and the same person in both areas.

- Challenge stereotypes in a *positive* and *creative* way. For example, talk to people rather than using email; generate an attitude of loving kindness toward others, all living things and yourself. This is about appreciating your social and natural environments.

- Move away from people who *drain* your energy: those that take your emotional and psychic energy but reciprocally give nothing back. This is not about avoidance, anger or blame on your part, this is about *disengagement*, literally meaning *you* let go of the emotional ties that bind you to that person or persons; this is about you reorganizing how you respond to them in such a way that you do not lose your precious energy resources when you are with them, but neither do you hurt them or do them harm.

- Do not *victimize* or *scapegoat* others, rather look for solutions and resolutions to difficulties and try to *understand* the other person rather than attribute blame. This is not easy, but if you can put yourself in the other person's shoes then you might just understand their situation a little a better.

Tame the email monster

This might seem a strange point to raise in a relational context, but think about it – you can get a deluge of mail on a daily basis; email is now one of the most important communication tools we have and can be invaluable in both work and social life. However, email respects no boundaries: in the technological age it is as available as the internet or mobile phone; it is your constant companion and you can spend an inordinate amount of time using email as a tool of communication. If you really think about it, you can be having several different conversations with several different people about several different things at any one moment in time. In one sense this can be time-saving; but the problem with multiple interchanges is that any one of those dialogues could be going awry because, when you are tired, exhausted and overloaded, the ability to receive or respond to the emotional and psychological content of the message in a meaningful and authentic way, can easily be misplaced.

Emails are *not* a method of face-to-face contact; they are a technological interface lacking verbal or non-verbal cues, except perhaps those we choose to add in 'cyber' speak. The problem with this kind of physical distance from the person you are talking to is that the relationship is sanitized; it is not real unless you mindfully make it so.

The solutions to managing the glut of mail you can receive and its boundary-less nature are manifold; most suggest a method of prioritizing your action, for example, act, read or ignore systems, others suggest answering emails at specific times. These may well work for you, but fundamentally you need to be mindful of and respond to others with feeling and with *emotional intelligence*: by focusing on the minutiae of the relational moment, really listening and responding, being present with the other and reciprocally respecting each other in the immediacy of moment in that dance of energy, so we can actually *live* the relationship.

CONCLUSION

When we feel, react and respond as human beings in action with, and as a result of, others in the same place, then the emotional exchange between us becomes reciprocal and *people*, rather than *task*, become the central context of what we do. If we could approach both the paid and unpaid workplace with a more caring, egalitarian and supportive attitude, then the notions of life balance that are held within that setting would become a by-product of those relational factors, and subsequently, so the theory goes, the approach to support imbalance can become one of nurture, not blame and it is the spirit of the network *itself* that becomes integral to the success of the workplace and life balance.

At times you can feel very impotent in an organization, but if you think in terms of interconnections, where each small step makes a change in other parts of the web, then however tiny that step may seem, you can and *do* make a difference to the bigger whole. In essence, life is not about performance, but meaning *and* connections. In your life, measure not just effectiveness and efficiency, but the impact you have on your own and other people's lives; it is this that is the real soul of a meaningful and balanced life.

CHAPTER 9
THE INTRICATE WEB OF LIFE BALANCE

INTRODUCTION

To conclude the book I would like to begin by thinking about what we have learned. Perhaps the biggest point is that harmony in life is not just about balancing the domains of work and life as much of the literature purports; life is much more complicated than this and is *multidimensional*, requiring a mutable and dynamic dance between a variety of doing, being, belonging and becoming activities, some of which must be engaging and personally meaningful in order to promote a sense of fulfillment and enjoyment in life. Life balance is about participating in relational networks from all walks of life, including appreciation of our connections with the natural environment, and it is this use of the human resources of time and energy that facilitates finding a congruent sense of self and is a doorway to personal wellbeing and developing a *meaning orientation* in life; it is this dynamic dance of time and energy that creates the intricate web of life balance (see Figure 9.1).

However, as I have mooted several times, this kind of interconnected model of life balance brings us back to the same old problem: in order to achieve a meaningful and harmonious lifestyle we have to value time and energy differently, and think about using these personally generated resources for participation in a variety of life activities, not just those considered obligatory or socially valued in whatever socio-cultural-political economy we are embedded. This means we have to adapt our thinking to reconcile, not compromise, our life balance.

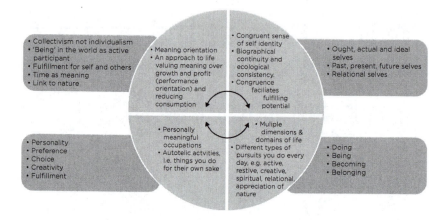

Figure 9.1 The intricate web of life balance

IF WE DO THIS WILL IT CHANGE?

If you adopt the strategies in the book and adapt your thinking then yes, you will achieve a personally meaningful sense of life balance. But the challenge remains that in a performance culture, resources, both human and environmental, are overused to sustain growth. As we reach the peak point of exhaustion in both elements, so we push more and more, and the spiral of intensification expands rather than detracting to achieve a sustainable point of balance or harmony. As long as we maintain a drive for wealth, growth and material consumption, namely, ride the cycles of productivity and consumerism, so that meaning-orientation necessary to achieve life balance remains latent.

The modern world gauges the success of nations through the rate of economic power and growth stimulated though productivity and consumerism, that is, the Gross Domestic Product (GDP). This tool wrongly assumes that human fulfillment and wellbeing is achieved through these quality indicators, and it pays little or no attention to the levels of human and natural resources that are used to achieve these ends, even though their depletion is directly related to life *imbalance* and their over-use challenges the sustainability and resilience of the social and environmental reserves for future generations.

The United Nations (UN) (2014) has tried to address some of these shortfalls and developed a second measure to supplement GDP called the Human Development Index (HPI). This identifies quality of life indicators as life expectancy, levels of education, and the standard of living measured through gross national income per capita. However, although more person-centered than the indices of the GDP, these indicators do not reflect the extant inequalities, or the levels of human security, safety, poverty and empowerment, in its scale. Consequently, it does little to identify the building blocks necessary for life balance, namely, autonomy, choice, meaning, personal empowerment, workers' rights and wellbeing, nor does it consider the over-consumption of human and natural resources utilized to promote growth, and therefore it has little relevance to the sustainability and resilience of human and environmental wellbeing, or indeed the search for meaning and fulfillment in life. So what are the alternatives?

MODELS OF SUSTAINABILITY AND RESILIENCE

Engagement with the natural environment has been proven to promote health, and there is a growing sense of awareness that human wellbeing is linked to the sustainability and resilience of not only the human resources held within people, but also those of the planet, with which we co-exist. O'Brien for example, identifies that sustainable human wellbeing is found in:

> Happiness that contributes to individual, community and/or global wellbeing without exploiting other people, the environment or future generations. This is aligned with the UN resolution on happiness and wellbeing and can be applied to individual lifestyles, community planning, national policies, and international agreements. (2013, pp.295–296)

Most of us, specifically in industrial and post-industrial societies, have long forgotten that we are an integral part of the ecosystem in which we live, and few of us have the time, energy or indeed inclination to spend time enjoying that. This is a sad indictment of contemporary ways of being and belonging in Western economies and worryingly, the long arm of global markets is now tainting all other cultures that wish to be part of, or have become entrapped in, that particular economic web. This kind of thinking and approach must be addressed if balance is to be fully realized in our lives and sustainability, resilience and a meaning orientation in life achieved at global levels.

The New Economics Foundation (NEF) (2006) has gone some way to addressing this by developing the Happy Planet Index (HPI) as a means to consider the ecological footprint of countries along with the lifespan and the subjective satisfaction of its people. That is to say, it considers the ecological efficiency of delivering human wellbeing and, as very few countries are doing well on this measure, the subsequent report is called the Unhappy Planet Index to reflect the gaping chasms these kinds of ecological consideration can illuminate.

Whilst the findings are not positive, this index is an excellent start to begin to recognize how the resources of the planet are finite and over-used. Moreover, querying subjective satisfaction does offer an opportunity to understand the health of the nation and how satisfied we, as people, actually feel individually and collectively about the quality of our lives; but the questions left hanging include those which consider whether we are happy 'enough' or if we are truly fulfilled in the sense of living a balanced and meaningful life.

As I have discussed previously in the book, one of the most insidious aspects of capitalism is that our sense of satisfaction can become skewed to socially meritorious goals rather than those associated with personal meaning and who we *really* are and *want* to become in life. Kahneman *et al.* (2006, p.1910) have called this capacity to absorb the things society says are good into our own drive for meaning as the 'focusing illusion'; the problem with this trap is that you may feel you are fulfilling your potential, but in reality you are lost in terms of your authentic purpose and meaning in life because you are walking the socially constructed 'ought' path:

> Despite the weak relation between income and global life satisfaction or experienced happiness, many people are highly motivated to increase their income. In some cases, this focusing illusion may lead to a misallocation of time, from accepting lengthy commutes (which are among the worst moments of the day) to sacrificing time spent socializing (which are among the best moments of the day). (Kahneman *et al.* 2006, p.1910)

In a world where the constant need for growth is associated with success and happiness, so we want more: the detached house, the posh car, those specific clothes or image and that fabulous holiday. To achieve this we work longer and harder, using more and more time and energy to generate the money to buy it; we also use more natural resources in order to feed and perpetuate the cycle of production in order to make the things we want to sell or buy. The problem, then, is that in a performance society driven by consumerism and consumption, individuals may mistakenly believe 'that "the goods life" is the path to "the good life"' (Kasser 2006, p.200) and in order to continue to produce 'stuff', over-use both human and natural resources to the point of exhaustion.

Yet wealth and symbolic capital does not sustain any greater happiness in the moment-by-moment experience for people; indeed it predisposes to higher levels of stress and ill-health (Kahneman *et al.* 2006). Alternatively, observing and nurturing supportive networks predicates long life and happiness (Xu and Roberts 2010) and being in and appreciative of the natural world sustains not only human but also ecological health and wellbeing (O'Brien 2013). To accomplish this vision of life balance we have to address our detachment from personal meaning and from the planet and, alternatively, observe and value the intricate connections of life balance. This means challenging the concept that paid work and material consumption are the *joie de vivre* of life, and seeking meaning and balance predicated in models of human and environmental resilience and sustainability. In essence, we must live and appreciate the ecology of life balance; that is far more essential to having a fulfilled and happy life and it is this that should be measured as our notion of success.

Whilst we wait for those in power to catch up and new economic models to flourish which put people and the planet before growth and money, we can, individually and collectively, make small moves. Box 9.1 offers a quick summary of the key messages in this book and a reminder of the ways you can practice these to realize and maintain *your* everyday life balance and the health and wellbeing of your relational networks and the natural environment.

Box 9.1 Key messages for achieving a sustainable, resilient life balance

Rediscover your sense of self

Recognize that the resilient and sustainable use of resources has to be the core of our lives

Do, be, belong, become and think of life as an interconnected whole

Be yourself and seek personal congruence and meaning

Engage in personally meaningful activities in life

Find a sense of meaning, engagement, joy and creativity in life

Value people over money and wellbeing over growth to achieve sustainable health and wellbeing in everyday life

Reclaim autonomy over your time and energy resources

Change the way you think; move from materialistic values and a performance orientation to one that is meaningful, more creative and innovative

Feed your psychic energy

Develop your imagination and experience flow

Value relationships and genuinely connect with others and the planet

See life balance as a complex, interconnected web

Recognize that links to nature are healing and sustain balance and wellbeing

Move from a performance to a meaning orientation

Exchange time not for money or growth but for meaning

Care for yourself, others, all living things and the planet

Make choices and reconcile, not compromise

Do meaningful things, engage, be creative, fulfill your potential and experience flow

Be mindful: Live in the moment

Support and live egalitarian and altruistic approaches to life balance

CONCLUSION

As the awareness of the interconnections between human wellbeing and the planet continues to grow, so the significance of this both individually and collectively has begun to seep into the unconsciousness and become more relevant in our everyday lives. As individuals, who are part of the greater whole, one thing we can do is spend more time in nature and find or re-establish our connections to it. Over time this will break down the illusion that money is of greater worth than wellbeing at an individual, collective and ecological level. In the interim, aim to live for meaning not performance; nurture relational networks and appreciate connections to the natural world; seek peace of mind and practice mindfulness; balance doing, being, becoming and belonging activities; come to know yourself and take the time to do the things you enjoy and love; do not compromise your personally meaningful and fulfilling pursuits for obligation and social credence, but rather choose to reconcile them, because your life balance is a journey of your own making and it can be fulfilling if you make it so. Last but not least, reconcile not compromise, simply because you are worth it.

GLOSSARY

Autonomy: Self-determination; ability to have free choice.

Becoming: 'Becoming' describes the idea that people can envision possible future selves and potentialities, achieve ideas about who and what they might want to become over time or through their lifespan, and attain a personal sense of congruence between who they want to be and who they do actually become.

Being: Appreciation of art and beauty, of life and contemplation; knowing who we are in terms of meaning; understanding and experiencing life moment by moment.

Being in the word: The sense of existing and experiencing being human in the world in relation to other things and the planet; linked to spirituality and existentialism, the search for meaning in life; recognizing the interconnected nature of life and our link to the planet as we exist in it.

Belonging: Sense of belonging is about relationships from everyday social interactions to more significant friendships, thus can encompass daily happenstances, workplace associations, social support networks and familial love and caring relationships. These kinds of social and personal encounters tend to be reciprocal, which means they meet our mutual needs for being cared for, loved, liked or valued by, and meaningful to, others. Belonging is also about having a *sense of place*, somewhere to settle, to be a part of and feel safe or secure in, and includes a recognition of belonging to the planet.

Biographical continuity: A continual sense of self-sameness (self-identity) across time.

Collectivism: Values social networks such as families, workplaces, societies and nations and sees the individual as only a part of that greater whole.

Doing: Purposeful, goal-oriented activities; also physically active occupations.

Domain: The sphere or area of activity in life.

Ecological consistency: Having a personal sense of coherence in one's behavior across different domains of life.

Emotional or subjective wellbeing: Refers to the presence of positive emotions as opposed to negative; it is about how we feel and subsequently, I would suggest, a personal sense of emotional wellbeing as opposed to the opposite, a sense of dis-ease or ill-being in everyday life.

Engagement: Focused psychic energy or attention to activity. Although experienced in meaningful occupation, this can be directed to make more mundane tasks interesting.

Ethical wellbeing: Living in an ethically sound way, which, in part, is measured by your congruence with the wider socially acceptable morals, values and behaviors that shape your culture. The paradox in Western constructs of work–life balance is that it creates moral and ethical dilemmas in terms of caring and paid work and erodes this type of wellbeing.

Flow: An experience of full engagement in an activity, where time disappears and you feel fully focused, absorbed and fulfilled. These types of experiences are known as 'optimal experiences'. See also 'Psychic energy'.

Individualism: Puts the rights of the individual before the group and values the inalienable right of the individual to live as he or she so chooses in terms of achieving personal goals, personal uniqueness, and personal control and marginalizing the social.

Intensification: Intensification, or in Paton's (2001, p.63) words a 'do more with less culture' which is redolent with increased workloads, work pressures and expectations and has become endemic in our paid work environments. As a consequence, workers experience pressure and stress, causing not only dissatisfaction and ill-health but significant life imbalance.

Locus of control: Center of control, which can be internal (self-determined) or external (controlled by an external agency or power separate to self).

Meaning: Something that is experienced as personally meaningful, that is, significant or important in an emotional and subjective sense.

Meaningful occupation: All occupations (activities) have a level of meaning because we respond to and interact with them, but in the context of this book meaningful occupation is meant to define a sense of fulfillment, a positive feeling/experience.

Meaning orientation: Reflects the extent to which personal and societal values are focused on something that is experienced as personally meaningful, that is, significant or important in a positive emotional and subjective sense. In this book the emphasis is on a connected relational context, seeking a meaningful life and personal fulfillment and consequently one's sense of spirituality and 'being in the world.'

Neoliberal/Neoliberalism: An economic model based on productivity, consumerism, consumption, individualism and profit.

Occupation/s: All the things we do every day.

Paid work: Your job, work or paid employment.

Performance orientation: Reflects the extent to which the employee is driven to meet organizational goals, standards, excellence, and performance improvement. It is supported by a workplace, culture or society driving personal responsibility, individualism, competiveness and materialism.

Personally meaningful: Something important and valued by you, usually the activities that you freely choose, enjoy, find pleasurable of fulfilling in life just for the sake of it. Finding time for these types of meaningful activity facilitates life balance.

Physical wellbeing: Refers to bodily health and function; it is how we feel physically.

Psychic energy: 'Attention' energy used to facilitate engagement and flow.

Psychological wellbeing: Refers to how we think, and importantly includes how we feel about our 'self', namely, our sense of self-acceptance, autonomy, personal growth and personal efficacy or mastery over a variety of life domains. Both the psychological and the emotional/subjective concepts encompass a sense of self-identity, personal congruence and coherence (consistency in knowing who I am) in everyday life.

Purposive: Something that serves or effects a useful function; the 'necessary' activities of life.

Rust-out: Apathy and/or disengagement from activities or life.

Self-responsibilization: An aspect of neoliberalism that places the members of society and consequently, the individual worker, as *personally responsible* for his or her own actions and therefore culpable for the consequences, intended or unintended. In terms of life balance this means the choice and decisions made to achieve work–life balance are the responsibility of the worker. In order to observe this shared notion of responsibility in the workplace, workers are subject to greater levels of scrutiny and control.

Sense of place: A sense of authentic human attachment to somewhere; also being in and belonging to the world or connection to the planet.

Sense of self: Knowing who I am; a congruent and coherent (consistent) self-identity and integrated multiple selves.

Significant other: Someone who is influential in your life or who has some emotional significance to you.

Social wellbeing: Is concerned with how we 'fit' with the social environment and is gauged by the contribution we give individually to society: this is about social capital, social worth and social acceptance by significant others. Notably, what is relevant about this in a sense of life balance and wellbeing is that one's level of success and self-worth is often a reflection of social values, norms and standards, so is a measure of how one meets the inherent expectations of the relevant social environment. Consequently, it is uniquely culturally defined, and your level of social integration, social contribution, social acceptance and social coherence is specific to your situated context.

Spiritual wellbeing: Considers, as indeed you may well think, both the religious and other more existential beliefs that encompass one's sense of purpose and/or direction in life and our sense of 'being' in the world. In essence, this is about who we are and who we want to be or become: our search for *meaning*, if you like, and living in congruence with the values we may hold.

Unpaid work: Obligatory tasks carried out in the non-paid work environment.

REFERENCES

Adam, B. (1995) *Timewatch: The Social Analysis of Time*. Cambridge: Polity Press.

Adam, B. (2003) 'Reflexive modernization temporalized.' *Theory, Culture and Society* 20, 2, 59–78.

Andersen, S.M. and Chen, S. (2002) 'The relational self: An interpersonal social-cognitive theory.' *Psychological Review 109*, 4, 619–645.

Beck, A.T. (1976) *Cognitive Therapy and the Emotional Disorders*. New York, NY: International Universities Press.

Beck, A.T., Rush, A.J., Shaw, B.F. and Emery, G. (1979) *Cognitive Therapy of Depression*. New York, NY: Guilford Press.

Berry, W. (2002) *The Art of the Commonplace*. Berkeley, CA: Counterpoint.

Bourdieu, P. (1989) 'Social space and symbolic power.' *Sociological Theory 71*, 1, 14–25.

Brannen, J. (2005) 'Time and the negotiation of work–family boundaries: Autonomy or Illusion.' *Time and Society 14*, 1, 113–131.

Brown, K.W. and Ryan, R.M. (2003) 'The benefits of being present: Mindfulness and its role in psychological well-being.' *Journal of Personality and Social Psychology 84*, 4, 822–848.

Bunting, M. (2005) *Willing Slaves: Why the Overwork Culture is Ruling our Lives*. London: Harper Collins.

Callan, S. (2007) 'Implications of family friendly policies for organizational culture: findings from two case studies.' *Work, Employment and Society 12*, 4, 673–691.

Capra, F. (1996) *The Web of Life: A New Synthesis of Mind and Matter*. London: Harper Collins.

Caproni, P.J. (2004) 'Work/life balance: You can't get there from here.' *Journal of Applied Behavioral Science 40*, 2, 208–218.

Carriere, J., Cheyne, A. and Smilek, D. (2008) 'Everyday attention lapses and memory failures: the affective consequences of mindlessness.' *Consciousness and Cognition 17*, 835–847.

Chaskalson, M. (2011) *The Mindful Workplace: Developing Resilient Individuals and Resonant Organizations*. Oxford: Wiley Blackwell.

Cheyne, J., Carriere, A. and Smilek, D. (2006) 'Absent-mindedness: Lapses of conscious awareness and everyday cognitive failures.' *Consciousness and Cognition 15*, 578–592.

Clark, S.C. (2000) 'Work/family border theory: A new theory of work/life balance.' *Human Relations 53*, 6, 747–770.

Clouston. T.J. (2014) 'Whose occupational balance is it anyway? The challenge of neoliberal capitalism and work-life imbalance.' *British Journal of Occupational Therapy 77*, 10, 507–515.

Coates, G. (1997) 'Organization man – Women and organizational culture.' *Sociological Research Online 2*, 3. Available at www.socresonline.org.uk/socresonline/2/3/7. html, accessed on 23 February 2015.

Costea, B., Crump, N. and Amiridis, K. (2008) 'Managerialism, the therapeutic habitus and the self in contemporary organizations.' *Human Relations 16*, 5, 661–685.

Coser, L. (1974) *Greedy Institutions: Patterns of Undivided Commitment.* New York, NY: Free Press.

Coyle, A. (2005) 'Changing Times: Flexibilization and the Re-organization of Work in Feminized Labor Markets.' In L. Pettinger, J. Parry, R. Taylor and M. Glucksmann (eds) *A New Sociology of Work?* Oxford: Blackwell.

Creek, J. (2003) *Occupational Therapy Defined as a Complex Intervention.* London: College of Occupational Therapists (COT).

Csikszentmihalyi, M. (1990) *Flow: The Psychology of Optimal Experience.* New York, NY: Harper Collins.

Csikszentmihalyi, M. (1997) *Finding Flow: The Psychology of Engagement with Everyday Life.* New York, NY: Harper Collins.

Csikszentmihalyi, M. (2002) *Flow: The Psychology of Happiness: The Classic Work on How to Achieve Happiness.* London: Rider.

Cummins, R.A. (1996) 'The domains of life satisfaction: An attempt to order chaos.' *Social Indicators Research 38*, 303–328.

Davidson, R.J. (2000) 'Affective style, psychopathology, and resilience: Brain mechanisms and plasticity.' *American Psychologist 55*, 11, 1192–1214.

Davidson S.J. (2010) 'Complex responsive processes: A new lens for the leadership on twenty-first-century health care.' *Nursing Forum 45*, 2, 108–117.

Diener, E. and Seligman, M.E.P. (2004) 'Beyond money: Toward an economy of well-being.' *Psychological Science in the Public Interest 5*, 1–31.

Dewe, P. and Kompier, M. (2008) *Foresight Mental Capital and Wellbeing Project. Wellbeing at Work: Future Challenges.* London: The Government Office for Science, HMSO.

Easwaran, E. (2008) *Passage Meditation: Bringing the Deep Mediation of the Heart into Daily Life,* 3rd edn. Tomales, CA: Nilgiri Press.

Edwards, D. and Burnard, P. (2003) 'A systematic review of the effects of stress and coping strategies used by occupational therapists working in mental health settings.' *British Journal of Occupational Therapy 66*, 8, 234–255.

Fidler, G. (1983) 'Doing and Becoming: The Occupational Therapy Experience.' In G. Kielhofner, (ed.) *Health Through Occupation: Theory and Practice in Occupational Therapy*. Philadelphia, PA: F.A. Davis.

Frankl, V. (2004) *Man's Search for Meaning*. Croydon: Rider Books.

Friedman, E.S., Thase, M.E. and Wright, M.E. (2008) 'Cognitive BehavioralTherapies.' In A. Tasman, K. Jerald, J.A. Lieberman, M.B. First, and M. Maj (eds) *Psychiatry*, 3rd edn. Chichester: John Wiley.

Gambles, R., Lewis S. and Rapoport, R. (2006) *The Myth of* Work-Life *Balance: The Challenge of our Time for Men, Women and Societies*. Chichester: John Wiley.

Gergen, K.J. (2000) *The Saturated Self: Dilemmas of Identity in Contemporary Life*. New York, NY: Basic Books.

Gershuny, J., Bittman, M. and Brice, J. (1997) '*Exit, Voice and Suffering: Do Couples Adapt to Changing Employment Patterns?*' Working Papers of the ESRC Research Centre on Micro-Social Change, Paper 97-8. Colchester: University of Essex.

Gershuny, J., Godwin, M. and Jones, S. (1994) 'The Domestic Division of Labor: a Process of Lagged Adaptation?' In M. Anderson, F. Bechhofer and J. Gershuny (eds) *The Social and Political Economy of the Household*. Oxford: Oxford University Press.

Gorz, A. (1980) *Farewell to the Working Class*. London: Pluto Press.

Greenhaus, J.H. (2008) 'Editorial Innovations in the study of the work–family interface: Introduction to the special section.' *Journal of Occupational and Organizational Psychology 81*, 343–348.

Grote, G. and Raeder, S. (2009) 'Careers and identity in flexible working: Do flexible identities fare better?' *Human Relations 62*, 2, 219–244.

Hakim, C. (2006) 'Women, careers and work-life preferences.' *British Journal of Guidance and Counselling 34*, 3, 279–294.

Hakim, C. (2007) Work-life *Choices in the 21st Century: Preference Theory*. Oxford: Oxford University Press.

Hammell, K.W. (2004) 'Dimensions of meaning in the occupations of daily life.' *Canadian Journal of Occupational Therapy 71*, 5, 296–305.

Hammell, K.W. (2011) 'Resisting theoretical imperialism in the disciplines of occupational science and occupational therapy.' *British Journal of Occupational Therapy 74*, 1, 27–33.

Handy, C. (1997) *The Hungry Spirit: Beyond Capitalism. A Quest for Purpose in the Modern World*. London: Hutchinson.

Hanh, T.N. (1991a) *Peace in Every Step*. London: Rider.

Hanh, T.N. (1991b) *Old Path White Clouds: Walking in the Footsteps of the Buddha*. Berkeley, CA: Parallax Press.

Hochschild, A. (2000) *The Time Bind: When Work Becomes Home and Home Becomes Work*, 2nd edn. New York, NY: Henry Holt.

Hochschild, A. (2008) 'On the Edge of the Time Bind: Time and Market Culture.' In C. Warhurst, R.E. Eikhof and A. Haunschild (eds) *Work Less, Live More? Critical Analysis of the Work–Life Boundary*. Basingstoke: Palgrave Macmillan, pp.80–91.

Holt, H. and Thaulow, I. (1996) 'Formal and In-formal Flexibility in the Workplace.' In S. Lewis and J. Lewis (eds) *The Work–Family Challenge. Rethinking Employment*. London: Sage, pp.79–92.

Kabat-Zinn, J. (1990) *Full Catastrophe Living: Using the Wisdom of your Body and Mind to Face Stress, Pain and Illness*. New York, NY: Delacourt.

Kahneman, D., Krueger, A.B., Schkade, D., Schwarz, N. and Stone, A.A. (2006) 'Would you be happier if you were richer? A focusing illusion.' *Science 312*, 1908–1910.

Kasser, T. (2006) 'Materialism and its Alternatives.' In M. Csikszentmihalyi and I.S. Csikszentmihalyi (eds) *A Life Worth Living*. Oxford: Oxford University Press.

Kimmel, S. (2009) 'Beyond volunteerism: Timebanking as a catalyst for community and economic regeneration.' *Social Policy 39*, 3, 4–9.

Kittay, E.F. (1999) *Love's Labor: Essays on Women, Equality and Dependency*. New York: Routledge.

Kofodimos, J. (1993) *Balancing Act: How Managers can Integrate Successful Careers and Fulfilling Personal Lives*. San Francisco, CA: Jossey-Bass.

Langer, E.J. (1992) 'Matters of mind: Mindfulness/mindlessness in perspective.' *Consciousness and Cognition 1*, 289–305.

Langer, E.J. (2014) 'Mindfulness in the age of complexity.' *Harvard Business Review*. Available at https://hbr.org/2014/03/mindfulness-in-the-age-of-complexity, accessed on 23 February 2015.

Lefebvre, H. (2004) *Rhythmanalysis*. London: Continuum.

Levitas, R. (2001) 'Against work: A utopian incursion into social policy.' *Critical Social Policy 21*, 4, 449–465.

Lloyd, C. and King, R. (2001) 'Work-related stress and occupational therapy.' *Occupational Therapy International 8*, 4, 227–243.

Mancini, M. (2003) *Time Management: 24 Techniques to Make Each Minute Count at Work*. New York, NY: McGraw-Hill Professional Education System.

Markus, H. and Nurius, P. (1986) 'Possible selves.' *American Psychologist 41*, 9, 954–969.

Maslow, A. (1954) *Motivation and Personality*. New York, NY: Harper.

Maslow, A. (1968) *Towards a Psychology of Being*, 3rd edn. New York, NY: John Wiley.

McDowell, L. (2004) 'Work, workfare, work/life balance and an ethic of care.' *Progress in Human Geography 28*, 145–163.

Mental Health Foundation (2003) *Whose Life is it Anyway? A Report on Poor Work–Life Balance on Mental Health*. London: Mental Health Foundation.

Meyer, A. (1922) The philosophy of occupation therapy. *Archives of Occupational Therapy 1*, 1, 1–10.

Meyerson, D. (2000) 'If Emotions were Honoured: A Cultural Analysis.' In S. Fineman (ed.) *Emotion in Organizations*. London: Sage.

Mindtools. (2003) Urgent and Important Matrix. Mindtools. Available at www.mindtools.com/pages/article/newHTE_91.htm, accessed on 23 February 2015.

Mintzberg, H., Ahlstrand, B. and Lampel, J. (1998) *The Strategy Safari*. Harlow: Pearson Education.

Muldoon, M.H. and King, J.N. (1991) 'A spirituality for the long haul: Response to chronic illness.' *Journal of Religion and Health 30*, 99–108.

Neenan, N. and Dryden, W. (2011) *Cognitive Therapy in a Nutshell*. London: Sage.

New Economics Foundation (NEF) (2006) *The Unhappy Planet Index*. London: NEF.

O' Brien, C. (2013) 'Who is teaching us about sustainable happiness and well-being?' *Health, Culture and Society 5*, 1, 294–307.

Odih, P. (2003) 'Gender, work and organization in the time/space economy of "Just-in-Time" labor.' *Time and Society 12*, 2/3, 293–314.

Paton, C. (2001) 'The state of health; Global capitalism, conspiracy, cock-up and competitive change in the NHS.' *Public Policy and Administration 16*, 4, 61–83.

Pawar, B.S. (2013) 'A proposed model of organizational behavior aspects for employee performance and well-being.' *Applied Research Quality Life 8*, 339–359.

Porter-O'Grady, T. and Malloch, K. (2003) *Quantum Leadership: A Textbook of New Leadership*. Sudbury, MA: Jones and Bartlett.

Praissman, S. (2008) 'Mindfulness-based stress reduction: A literature review and clinician's guide.' *Journal of the American Academy of Nurse Practitioners 20*, 212–216.

Putnam, R. (2000) *Bowling Alone: The Collapse and Revival of American Community*. New York, NY: Simon and Schuster.

Ransome, P. (2008) 'The Boundary Problem in Work–Life Balance.' In C. Warhurst, R.E. Eikhof and A. Haunschild (eds) *Work Less, Live More? Critical Analysis of the Work-Life Boundary*. Basingstoke: Palgrave Macmillan, pp.62–79.

Rebeiro, K.L., Day, D., Semeniuk, B., O'Brien, M. and Wilson, B. (2001) 'Northern initiative for social action: An occupation based mental health program.' *American Journal of Occupational Therapy 55*, 493–500.

Reiter, N. (2007) 'Work–life balance: What DO you mean? The ethical ideology underpinning appropriate application.' *Journal of Applied Behavioral Science 43*, 273–294.

Rogers, C. (1961) *A Therapist's View of Psychotherapy: On Becoming a Person*. Wiltshire: Constable.

Rowles, G.D. (1991) 'Beyond performance: Being in place as a component of occupational therapy.' *American Journal of Occupational Therapy 45*, 265–271.

Sapolsky, R. (2004) *Why Zebras Don't get Ulcers*. London: Henry Holt Publishers.

Schaef, A. (2004) *Meditations for Women Who Do Too Much*. Revised edition. New York, NY: Harper Collins.

Scharmer, C.O. (2006). 'Theory U: Leading from the future as it emerges. The social technology of presenting.' *Fieldnotes* September/October, 1–13.

Schumacher, E.F. (1979) *Good Work*. (published posthumously). Available at www.scribd.com/doc/563164/Goodwork-EF-Schumacher, accessed 23 February 2015.

Sennett, R. (1998) *The Corrosion of Character: The Personal Consequences of Working the New Capitalism*. New York: WW Norton.

Sevenhuijsen, S. (2000) 'Caring in the third way: the relations between obligation, responsibility and care in third way discourse.' *Critical Social Policy 20*, 1, 5–37.

Stebbins, R.A. (2004) *Between Work and Leisure: The Common Ground of Two Separate Worlds*. New Brunswick: Transaction Publishers.

Stoll, R. (1989) 'The Essence of Spirituality.' In V. Carson (ed.) *Spiritual Dimensions of Nursing Practice*. Philadelphia, PA: WB Saunders.

Strati, A. (1992) 'Aesthetic understanding of organizational life.' *Academy of Management Review 17*, 3, 568–581.

Thompson, J.A. and Bunderson, J.S. (2001) 'Work–nonwork conflict and the phenomenology of time.' *Work and Occupations 38*, 1, 17–39.

Tolle, E. (2005) *The Power of Now: A Guide to Spiritual Enlightenment*. London: Hodder.

Townsend, E. (1997) 'Occupation: potential for personal and social transformation.' *Journal of Occupational Science 4*, 1, 18–26.

United Nations Development Programme (2014) *Human Development Index*. Human Development Reports: United Nations Development Programme. Available at http://hdr.undp.org/en/content/human-development-index-hdi, accessed on 23 February 2015.

Urry, J. (1995) *Consuming Places*. London: Routledge.

Watson, J. (2003) 'Love and caring: Ethics of face and hand – an invitation to return to the heart and soul of nursing and our deep humanity.' *Nursing Administration Quarterly 27*, 3, 197–202.

Wheatley, M.J. (1999) *Leadership and the New Science: Discovering Order in a Chaotic World*. San Francisco, CA: Berrett Koehler.

Wilcock, A.A. (1999) 'Reflections on doing, being and becoming.' *Australian Journal of Occupational Therapy 46*, 1–11.

Woolliams, P. and Trompenaars, F. (2013) 'Realizing change through other ways of working: Reconciling competing demands.' *Organization Development Journal 31*, 2, 6–16.

Xu, J. and Roberts, R.E. (2010) 'The power of positive emotions: It's a matter of life or death – Subjective well-being and longevity over 28 years in a general population.' *Health Psychology 29*, 9–19.

SUBJECT INDEX

AUTHOR INDEX